CONTENTS

Abbreviations

Introduction: Iain McCalman — i

Part One: Communication—Media Scares, Moral Panics, and Government Responses

Cathy Banwell and Charles Guest
  Carnivores, Cannibals, Consumption and Unnatural Boundaries: The BSE—CJD epidemic in the Australian press — 3

Michael Fitzpatrick
  How Now Mad Cow? — 37

Part Two: Science and Social Science— Evaluating Risks

Colin L. Masters
  Creutzfeldt-Jakob Disease: Rare transmissible spongiform encephalopathy with an important message — 71

Simon Grant
  Risk Assessment and Creutzfeldt-Jakob Disease — 83

Part Three: Humanities—Histories, Pathologies and Poetics

Harriet Ritvo
    The Roast Beef of Old England   97

Hank Nelson
    Kuru: The pursuit of the prize
      and the cure   125

Robin Wallace-Crabbe
    Mad Cow Disease: A bovine viewpoint   167

Contributors   187

MAD COWS AND MODERNITY

Cross-disciplinary Reflections on the Crisis
of Creutzfeldt-Jakob Disease

MAD COWS AND MODERNITY

Cross-disciplinary Reflections on the Crisis of Creutzfeldt-Jakob Disease

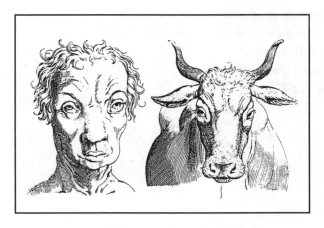

De Humana Physionomia (Naples, 1586)

edited by Iain McCalman with Benjamin Penny and Misty Cook

Humanities Research Centre, The Australian National University
National Academies Forum
1998

Humanities Research Centre Monograph Series No. 13
The Australian National University, Canberra ACT 0200
ISBN No. 0-7315-3305-4
First Published 1998
Copyright © 1998

Printed in Australia by Goanna Print, Fyshwick, Canberra

ABBREVIATIONS

BSE	Bovine Spongiform Encephalopathy
CJD	Creutzfeldt-Jakob Disease
GDP	Gross Domestic Product
MAFF	Ministry of Agriculture, Fisheries and Food
nvCJD	New variant form of Creutzfeldt-Jakob Disease
PrP	Prion Protein
PrP^C	The normal isoform of PrP
PrP^{SC}	The scrapie isoform of PrP
PRNP	The gene for PrP
SEAC	Spongiform Encephalopathy Advisory Committee
TSE	Transmissible Spongiform Encephalopathy
WHO	World Health Organization

INTRODUCTION

The cattle disease now known as Bovine Spongiform Encephalopathy (BSE), or popularly Mad Cow Disease, was first reported in Britain on 25 April 1985.[1] In Australia that was Anzac Day, an annual day of commemoration and mourning for citizens who had died in war. To British citizens it carried no such significance, yet it is tempting to see this moment as portentous, for the anxieties and heartbreaks that lay ahead were not unlike casualties of war. And for British farmers the veterinary report that a cow in Kent named Daisy had died after exhibiting odd dementia-like symptoms presaged an unimaginable slaughter of livestock and destruction of livelihood. But the critical moment when an economic and livestock disaster transformed itself into a crisis of humanity occurred on 20 March 1996 at which time the House of Commons was told of startling recent medical evidence from a group of Edinburgh-based specialists. The work of Dr Robert Will and his colleagues appeared to confirm long-festering fears that the cattle disease BSE had managed to jump the chasm of the species to infect humans, producing a new strain of Transmissible Spongiform Encephalopathy (TSE) now dubbed a new variant form of Creutzfeldt-Jakob Disease (nvCJD).[2] From that moment Creutzfeldt-Jakob Disease (CJD), previously a subject of relatively esoteric medical research, became the source of a global media frenzy and moral panic. Almost overnight Mad Cow Disease became a household phrase and thereafter rapidly gave rise to a spate of articles, books, seminars, research grants, inquiries, satirical sketches, and ghoulish jokes.

Such a panic had not been altogether predictable. The range and depth of feeling generated clearly took many government officials by surprise.

They were not alone in this: some experts in the sciences and social sciences also thought, and perhaps still think, that the popular outcry was disproportionate to the risks of acquiring what was after all a rare medical condition. Yet the idea of Mad Cow Disease undoubtedly struck some deep psychic chord amongst peoples of the western world in particular. Within the sphere of culture it took on an almost feral life of its own. Mad cows appeared in everything from avant-garde painting to children's computer games. A notable feature of much of the cultural, as distinct from specialist, commentary on the BSE and CJD crisis was its universalist and apocalyptic resonance. Popular analysts persistently implied that the disease was somehow representative of a larger social pathology, a disease of the human condition. Links and analogies with the earlier HIV/AIDS scare were legion. Moral lessons were everywhere adduced: here was another instance of nemesis provoked not so much by promiscuity as by our arrogance, greed, and wholesale abuse of nature. The disease's mysterious protein-like form (prions), irrational behavioural symptoms, long and covert gestation, and entanglement with political-economic as well as scientific-commercial agendas made it a supremely fruitful source for media punditry. In short, Mad Cow Disease quickly attained the relatively rare status of a global populist issue. Even now it continues to fascinate, grip and frighten people of all ages, genders, and walks of life, and from every corner of the world. It has become an icon of our time.

The severity of the crisis posed by BSE and CJD is one simple justification for publishing this book, but it is by no means the sole one. Other voices have been raised on the issue, and other surveys of the leading events have been written. We cannot even claim to be producing the first analysis from an Australian perspective: one of the best and most recent general studies *Cannibals, Cows, and the CJD Catastrophe,* happens to have come from an Australian science journalist, Jennifer Cooke. Of course we believe that our book, which gathers an exceptionally talented and diverse group of experts from Australia, Britain and the United States to deploy their specialized medical, social and cultural skills, will contribute fresh insights to an immensely complex story. But we are also seeking to do something else which we believe has not been attempted by any other publication dealing with this crisis. Our book aims particularly to address one feature of the BSE/CJD tragedy which has attracted a good deal of passing comment but no action. We draw attention to, and at the same time work to remedy, the fact that the segregation or isolation of experts actually exacerbated the BSE/CJD disaster. Professional competitiveness, intellectual parochialism, and institutional jealousies amongst specialists, scholars, and policy makers undoubtedly contributed to the relatively slow or inappropriate diagnoses and remediation of both BSE and nvCJD. The fragmentation and hyper-specialization of modern knowledge, a perceptible tendency in the west from at least the eighteenth century, has undoubtedly become one of the leading problems of our time. Arguably it is this that has given rise to the pervasive late twentieth-century cultural paradigm of postmodernity: if we cannot know something in a deep and holistic way we must shape our meanings from shards. But even militant postmodernists regret intellectual dessication and would probably join the authors of this book in stressing the importance of cross–disciplinary dialogue and exchange.

Early in 1996, around the same time as the BSE/CJD bombshell was exploding in Britain, a group of officials from the four Australian learned academies met informally to express their concern over such disciplinary divides among our scholars and, still more, over diminishing government support for scholarly research of all kinds. Out of this meeting came a new organization, called the National Academies Forum, comprising selected office bearers from the Academies of Science, Social Sciences, Humanities, and Technology. It aimed to work as a lobby group to ginger government, as a coordinating body to formulate policy advice for all four academies, and as a catalyst for encouraging intellectual dialogue across our various disciplinary and institutional chasms. When Professor Paul Bourke, President of the Academy of the Social Sciences in Australia, and Professor Sir Gustav Nossal, President of the Australian Academy of Science, were casting around over the dinner table for a suitable subject with which to launch this cross-academy dialogue, and which would engage the common intellectual interest of their diverse constituency, they lit on the inspiration of the BSE and CJD crisis. Here was an issue surely in which most Academy members would have both a specialized and a general interest. I was asked to help arrange, at the Humanities Research Centre of the Australian National University, a small one-day colloquium designed mainly for National Academies Forum and Academy members, but open to any other interested persons who wished to attend. Professor Nossal provided us with one of the world's leading CJD medical researchers from Melbourne University; Professor Bourke provided two distinguished scholars in economics and in social history from the Institute of Advanced Studies at the Australian National University, and I provided one of the University's Creative Arts Fellows, a celebrated painter, writer, and cattleman.

Although these contributors were given very short notice and the program was near spontaneous in its contrivance, the result of this colloquium proved to be genuinely inspirational. Both the subject of 'Mad Cows and Modernity' and the extraordinary diversity of approaches amongst the paper presenters seemed to rivet the audience. I have had to mount scores of scholarly conferences over the past five years, but I can recall none that generated such a palpable sense of enthusiasm and excitement. Discussion and debate among the audience turned out to be as searching, wide-ranging and informed as among the paper presenters; members of each academy seemed intrigued and sometimes astonished at the kind of work being conducted by counterparts in other fields. As well as engaging with the gripping and sometimes grim contents of the papers, discussants commented on the very different ways in which intellectual problems were posed, treated and presented by those in other disciplines. No-one seemed to want the colloquium to end and two morals were drawn over and over again: first, it was thought imperative that we bring our research out of specialist enclaves and engage regularly in this type of cross-disciplinary dialogue; second, it was agreed that we needed to make the contents of this particular colloquium public. The subject was too important and the implications of the papers too portentous to let lie. So, after I had commissioned a further three articles from experts in media analysis and science history from Australia, Britain and the United States, the jointly-sponsored Humanities Research Centre and National Academies Forum book *Mad Cows and Modernity: Cross-disciplinary reflections on the crisis of Creutzfeldt-Jakob disease* came into being.

The book is divided into three broad sections, and we have deliberately preserved the diverse styles, protocols, and referencing conventions preferred by each of the different disciplines represented. Our aim is to represent disciplinary difference within an overall unity of purpose. Part one gathers two articles located broadly within the modern intellectual field of Communication to reflect on media scares, moral panics, and governmental responses aroused by the BSE/CJD crisis. In 'Carnivores, Cannibals, Consumption and Unnatural Boundaries'

Iain McCalman

Cathy Banwell and Charles Guest, both researchers at the Australian National University's National Centre for Epidemiology and Population Health, survey a large sample of the Australian daily and specialist press to chart the shifting miasma of concerns raised by the crisis over time. They show how the relative distance of Australia from the centre of the crisis in Britain lent an apparently greater air of objectivity to Australian commentary, at least initially. Yet we began to generate our own versions of media scaremongering and moral panic through the importation of foreign journalism, combined with a growing realization that Australia was not in fact immune from either the economic or medical ramifications of BSE/CJD, particularly when the horrifying effects of infected growth hormone began to emerge. And although Banwell and Guest do not say so explicitly, it seems likely that we have still to reap the longterm consequences of using infective pituitaries for fertility programs and performance enhancement in sport and body building during the 1970s and 1980s. It would be a sad irony if CJD began to surface amongst the elite sportsmen and women at the 2000 Olympics in Sydney.

Both chapters in this section explore the actions and implications of moral panics, a concept pioneered by media analyst and sociologist Stanley Cohen in the 1960s. As with the hysteria over AIDS, they argue, deep-seated social taboos and culturally constructed moral boundaries were implicated in the public response to the transmissible spongiform 'epidemic'. Cannibalistic interferences with the food chain or enhancements of our genetic endowments were felt to be transgressions of the natural order which produced a cosmic retribution. Banwell and Guest also dissect some of the key narrative conventions and rhetorical strategies which helped shape the way that medical, social, political and economic reportage was presented and interpreted in Australia and abroad. Conceding that press and public have long been susceptible to such periodic outbreaks of moral panic on taboo issues, our second contributor Michael Fitzpatrick, a leading British medical practitioner and writer, nevertheless argues that much of the hysteria in Britain was whipped up needlessly by inept government responses to the media. In his chapter 'How Now Mad Cow' Fitzpatrick shows that clumsy or evasive press releases dealing with potentially combustible news served to inflame popular fears and precipitated a series of reactive governmental policies which were either purely cosmetic or grossly out of proportion to the actual public risk involved.

'Evaluating Risk' is the overarching theme of Part two which contains two chapters working from within the cognate, if distinct, perspectives and methodologies of the natural and social sciences. Colin L. Masters, Professor of Pathology at the University of Melbourne and one the world's foremost authorities on TSEs surveys the medical history and current experimental findings on the links between BSE and nvCJD. A model of brevity, clarity and rigour, his summation comes from the very cutting edge of medical knowledge. Its technical vocabulary in no way masks the urgency of the 'important message' that Masters spells out with characteristic restraint: 'While the bovine disease appears to be coming under control, a very large question mark hangs over the future extent of the spread of this disease into the human population'. Yet how should that human population respond to the risk of contracting CJD in everyday life? How are we to evaluate the degree of risk attached to the consumption of beef and beef products, particularly in Britain? Simon Grant, Professor of Economics at the Australian National University, shows us how specialists in social risk assessment evaluate questions such as this. Deploying a body of 'rational choice theory', or more properly 'non-subjective expected utility theory', that is commonly used by economists, he comes up with conclusions that are sometimes surprising and paradoxical. Apparent over-reactions in government policy, for example, can be driven by a valid and often effective logic, such as the need to restore fragile public confidence and trust after it has been overwhelmed by an almost unstoppable public opinion cascade.

The historical and cultural roots of such public opinion movements are the subject of the engrossing opening essay of the third and final section of the book where the histories, pathologies and poetics of the mad cow crisis are analysed by three diverse scholars and practitioners of the humanities. Harriet Ritvo, Arthur J. Conner Professor of History at the Massachusetts Institute of Technology, shows in her chapter, 'The Roast Beef of Old England', how eating beef became deeply ingrained within the British national psyche from the early eighteenth century when the country was experiencing both industrial modernity and global imperial expansion. No wonder, then, that an insidious disease apparently conveyed by that self-same British beef in the late twentieth century at a time of perceived national decline should hurt the British people and press so deeply. Yet the most palpable and horrifying consequences of the new spongiform encephalopathies were actually experienced not in Britain but across the other side of the world in the remote Highlands region of New Guinea. In 'Kuru: The pursuit of the prize and the cure', Hank Nelson, Professor of History in the Research School of Pacific and Asian Studies of the Australian National University, crafts a history of the tragic decimation of the Fore people of New Guinea by a mysterious shaking dementia they called Kuru. Nelson's haunting story of how the obsessed medical genius Carleton Gajdusek described the disease and eventually linked it to a long-lapsed practice of cannibalism has all the adrenalin-inducing properties of an

Oscar-winning film epic. But Australians have cause for some self-scrutiny as well, as Nelson deftly reveals the linkages between Kuru and our colonial endeavours, and gently points out the multiple and cross-disciplinary contributions underlying the sensational 'discovery' which earned Gajdusek a Nobel Prize.

Finally and fittingly our last chapter returns to where the story began, with a horrible disease that appeared to drive cows mad. Robin Wallace-Crabbe, Australian artist, novelist, art critic, raconteur, and farmer offers us an exuberant, witty, and characteristically original analysis of Mad Cow Disease largely from the viewpoint of the cow. Combining autobiography, discursive digression, linguistic pyrotechnics, and sheer technical know-how, his essay arrests, inverts and humanizes the crisis in a manner reminiscent of the great nineteenth-century essayist William Hazlitt. It is in the nature of the essayist and the artist to be able to reveal the world in a grain of sand; Wallace-Crabbe engages our humanity, finally, with a simple visual supplement to his chapter. A wonderfully sane and gentle cow (or is it a bull?) stands in an Australian paddock staring ruefully into the distance. Could this be an antipodean Daisy captured in paint at the moment before the affliction strikes, sensing the insanity of the human race from whom no barbed wire fence can protect her?

Iain McCalman

NOTES

[1] Jennifer Cooke, *Cannibals, Cows and the CJD Catastrophe: Tracing the shocking legacy of a twentieth century disease* (Sydney: Random House, 1998), p.117.

[2] Cooke, *Cannibals ...*, pp. 292-300.

Part One

Communication:
Media Scares, Moral Panics, and Government Responses

CARNIVORES, CANNIBALS, CONSUMPTION AND UNNATURAL BOUNDARIES: THE BSE—CJD EPIDEMIC IN THE AUSTRALIAN PRESS

Cathy Banwell and Charles Guest

INTRODUCTION

The complex saga of BSE in cattle and its possible links with nvCJD has aroused deep public concern. The media played a central role in informing the public about events as they unfolded and offered multiple meanings and interpretations. We take the BSE and nvCJD saga, as represented in three Australian newspapers, to consider the relationship between science, the media and public health.

METHOD

On 20 March 1996 the British government acknowledged that, despite previous statements to the contrary, a possible link existed between BSE, which was widespread in British cattle herds, and a newly discovered form of CJD in humans. In Britain, and indeed around the world, this admission ignited widespread press interest. This chapter analyses the resulting press coverage in *The Australian, The Sydney Morning Herald* and *The Australian Financial Review* for the first half of 1996. Any articles published in the last two papers which contained a reference to Mad Cow Disease, were downloaded from the 'ERIC' CD ROM data base. *The Australian*'s articles on Mad Cow Disease were obtained from a staff member of the paper. Further reports were obtained from a range of journals including *Scientific American, The Bulletin, The Economist, Time, Nature* and *Science*. These, and academic articles on risk, the media, Mad Cow Disease, and epidemics, informed the theoretical analysis.

The Data Set

The Sydney Morning Herald covered the events with a range of articles, many written by journalists located in the United Kingdom, Europe and America (thirty-two) and fewer produced locally (eighteen). Most overseas articles were reports on the story as a series of recent news events while a smaller number (nine) contained a mix of this style of reporting and commentary on the social, political and economic implications. Australian journalists for *The Sydney Morning Herald* also employed both forms of coverage. Those located in Australia covered the actions of local officials in response to the British findings and the implications of the events in Britain for Australians as consumers and producers of beef. A further thirteen articles in *The Sydney Morning Herald* by Australia-based journalists took the form of commentaries on the BSE and nvCJD saga. Several of these were lengthy and detailed pieces offering explanations and causes of the diseases as well as an overview of the progress of the affair in Britain. During the period until end of June another thirty-four pieces in *The Sydney Morning Herald* contained references to BSE and nvCJD and related topics. Roughly half were letters to the paper on the subject and the remainder consisted of mainly brief, and often humourous, comments.

The Australian's coverage on the story also derived from a mix of articles originating from overseas (fourteen news items and nine commentaries) and locally, (twenty-one news items and twenty-six commentaries). It used fewer articles accessed directly from overseas news services, such as *Reuters*, or overseas papers. A number of articles were written by *The Australian's* correspondents located overseas. It too printed letters and brief humorous comments on the topic.

For *The Australian Financial Review* the BSE and nvCJD story was a crisis of markets and economics rather than public health. Over the same period (until 30 June 1996) it contained twenty-two articles referring to BSE and nvCJD or related topics. Seven articles were written by *The Australian Financial Review* journalists located overseas, with the majority coming from their London-based correspondent. Six articles by Australian-based journalists were news reports on the impact of BSE on the Australian beef industry, while a further two articles were commentaries, one of them on the Australian food industry. Another five articles contained mainly brief and humorous references to the Mad Cow Disease.

REPORTING OF THE SEQUENCE OF EVENTS OF THE BSE EPIDEMIC AND THE nvCJD OUTBREAK

The story of BSE and nvCJD was presented as an unfolding of events over time (Ellingsen 1996; Woolford 1996; anon 1996c) in a number of articles from both overseas and Australian sources. This form of presentation strengthened the impact of BSE and nvCJD as a narrative with political, policy and moral messages. Although the causes of nvCJD are still undetermined, it was frequently reported as a chain of events commencing with the human actions that were considered to be responsible for initiating the problem. Thus, the inclusion of specific events, which were covered in several articles as follows, was a highly political choice.

Policy Background in the United Kingdom

One article commenced with a description of the British Thatcher government's abandonment of proposals in 1979 to prevent cattle being fed sheep meat potentially contaminated with scrapie, a long-standing spongiform encephalopathy (Ellingsen 1996). Other articles cited 1981 as the beginning of the disaster when deregulation of the feed industry to reduce costs allowed ruminant feed to be prepared at lower temperatures than was used previously. It is now suspected that this change allowed the supposed causative agents, prions, to be transmitted to cattle in feed; thus producing BSE (Radford 1996).

BSE first appeared in 1985 but it was not until the following year that the pathology was recognized and named.[1] It became a notifiable disease in 1988 when it was announced that infected cows would be destroyed. In the same year Australia banned the import of British cattle while Britain itself banned the consumption of offal including brain and spinal cord in 1989. The following year a host of European, and other countries banned live cattle imports from Britain and, in some cases, British cattle products such as milk. The British Minister for Agriculture denied risks of human infection from BSE and in a public demonstration for the media fed a hamburger to his four year old daughter. *The Lancet* reported on a death from nvCJD in a farm worker which was linked with BSE in 1993 (anon 1996c). Two years later, a group of 'eminent scientists' reported that they had stopped eating British beef (Ellingsen 1996); in the same year, Britain banned the inclusion of spinal column in 'mechanically recovered' meat.

In September 1995 the United Kingdom CJD Surveillance Unit first examined tissue samples from young patients with unusual CJD characteristics. By the end of February 1996, the CJD unit had eight cases of what appeared to be a new strain of CJD. An urgent meeting of the Spongiform Encephalopathy Advisory Committee (SEAC) was held on 8 March. By the time the committee met again on 16 March and then again on 18 March a further two cases had been discovered. On 20 March the British government announced that there may be a link between BSE and CJD (anon 1996e).

The citing of the Thatcher government's intervention in 1979 and the deregulation of the feed industry in 1981, implicated the government in the development of the epidemic of nvCJD in humans. This theme, taken up in other articles, focused on the Tory government's management of BSE and particularly that of Ministry of Agriculture, Fisheries and Food (MAFF). This body was roundly criticized for being influenced by the farm lobby, for not doing more to control BSE, and for denying the possibility of a link with human disease (anon 1996d). It was perceived to be secretive and have a 'bureaucratic fetish' for controlling the flow of information on BSE and CJD. Parkinson, writing for *The Australian*, reported that MAFF attempted to 'isolate' and 'vilify' scientists who argued that the government was underestimating the risks. He argued that scientific caution about risks allowed the British government to act as if there were no risk (Parkinson 1995). These statements were later reiterated in an editorial in the issue of *The Lancet* containing the report on the new cases of CJD. The editor (anon 1996b) attacked the 'secretive and inadequate way in which government ministers garner their expert advice'.

The government was also criticized for ignoring the practice of fattening cattle with bonemeal, brains and offal from dead cattle (Parkinson 1995). Furthermore, it was noted that farmers were not paid full compensation for the slaughter of their BSE infected cattle until 1990 which scarcely encouraged compliance with requirements of the cull.

The release of statements by the British government about a possible link between BSE and nvCJD before the publication of the relevant scientific paper was considered inept. The government's statement was made on 20 March 1996 and the paper published in *The Lancet* on 6 April (Will, Ironside et al. 1996) provoked complaints within the scientific community that they could not assess the science on which the claims were made (anon 1996b). Thus, the British government was attacked for its management of BSE and its links with nvCJD. The press coverage's most consistent and widespread criticisms were those of secrecy and the denial of any risk.

Australian Public Health Action

The BSE and nvCJD saga and its implications for Australian beef consumers, as reported in the press was markedly simpler, shorter and less contested than in Britain. As Australia had not imported fresh or frozen beef from Britain for many years, and had, since 1988, prohibited the importation of live cattle, cattle semen and cattle embryos, the country was reported to be safe from BSE. The day after the British government's announcement, Australia's National Food Authority requested information from the Australian Food Council on all foods which may have contained British beef (Hoy and Cooke 1996).

An emergency meeting was held on 22 March 1996 involving members of government departments and expert groups. The following day a taskforce was set up to recommend and coordinate the Australian response to the BSE and nvCJD crisis. The taskforce established a national communications strategy for use during an outbreak of an emerging or exotic disease, including the establishment of a telephone line, to answer questions about BSE and nvCJD and the safety of beef products in Australia.

On 26 March, a public statement was made by Primary Industries and Energy Minister, Mr John Anderson, and Health and Family Services Minister, Dr Michael Wooldridge, concerning the establishment of the task force. They announced that there was no BSE in Australian cattle, Australian beef was safe to eat, and that an investigation of foods available in Australia which contained British beef products would be made. Several days later, five products believed to contain British beef were withdrawn from sale. The stock feed industry in Australia, followed the World Health Organization (WHO) recommendations by voluntarily banning the feeding of meat and bone meal (including blood meal sourced from ruminants) to other ruminant animals (BSE/CJD Scientific Advisory Group 1996). This ban was later enforced through legislation (Beale 1996).

Media Response to Australia's Actions on BSE and nvCJD

An article on the 23 March in *The Sydney Morning Herald* (Hoy and Cooke 1996) reported on the investigation into the safety of beef products imported from Britain, including Marmite, Bovril and 'even chocolate'. In it, Australia's Dr Tony Adams, Chief Medical Adviser for the Commonwealth Department of Health and Family

Services, was quoted as saying that no milk products could be 'ruled out as being totally free from the cattle disease'. The article discussed all areas of identified risk, such as contaminated foods, and other beef products (makeup, live beef imports and semen). Dr Adams added, 'Hopefully, people won't be panicked'.

Subsequently, brief articles appeared in the papers reporting, for example, that 'Bovril [is] Safe' and that 'there is minimal risk from most manufactured foods from BSE in Australia' (anon 1996h). They advised the removal of products containing British beef from supermarket shelves and the announcement of a strategy to deal with the European Union's decision to ban British beef. Australians who had visited the United Kingdom in the high risk period from 1981 to 1989 were told that their risk was slight given the small number of cases of nvCJD. A toll-free telephone number, established by the taskforce, was published for inquiries about food products (Stott 1996).

The media's response to the Australian government's action on BSE and nvCJD and its impact was muted. The implications of the diseases for Australia received less attention in the Australian media than the more dramatic events in the United Kingdom and Europe. In articles, originating both locally and overseas, the attention was shifted from the putative link between BSE and nvCJD to the impact on the British beef market of the European Union ban, and its likely effect on the Australian beef industry. The Australian media's acceptance of statements about low, but acknowledged, risks to Australian consumers offered a contrast to the highly politicized and suspicious response in the British media to official statements about

BSE and nvCJD. However, the British press was responding not only to concerns about the safety of British beef but also to the occurrence of other food scares during the previous ten years.

A number of articles raised, with reference to BSE and nvCJD, the importance of safeguarding the standards of the Australian meat and food industry, and recent outbreaks of food contamination (Cribb 1996). Broader responses, exemplified by an editorial in *The Australian*, commented upon the fragility of food markets in the face of loss of consumer confidence and the need for continued care with quality-control and inspection (anon 1996).

The media coverage, exemplified by *The Australian* and *The Sydney Morning Herald*, of Australian official responses to BSE and nvCJD was not alarmist. While reporters felt that it was difficult to get a prompt government response when the story first broke, they were eventually satisfied with official statements that there was little risk to Australian consumers. From the government's side it was considered important to provide easy access to information (via the media and the telephone information line), to prevent the release of contradictory information and to acknowledge that there were risks involved, although small. Tony Adams later expressed the view that ' ... the co-ordinated media liaison between the various government agencies ... helped ensure a balanced and measured reporting of our BSE and nvCJD efforts by the Australian media' (BSE/CJD Scientific Advisory Group 1996). It is not possible to say whether the government's media strategy would have been as effective if BSE had been discovered in Australia.

THE SOCIAL, CULTURAL AND HISTORICAL CONTEXTS REFLECTED IN THE PRESS

Press coverage drew upon broader social, cultural and political contexts to explain the unfolding story of BSE, its putative link with nvCJD and to draw lessons from it. We examined the use of language and metaphor in this coverage, and the way in which they referred to these broader contexts.

Three interrelated explanatory themes of consumption, unnatural practices, and breached boundaries, appeared in accounts of BSE and nvCJD. Consumption, in particular, is central to many of these narratives. Though the link remains unproven, and there have been concerns that CJD may be contracted through other forms of contact with cattle, consumption was the major focus of press coverage as an explanation of BSE and CJD.

'We have turned vegetarian cows into carnivores and then into cannibals' one expert is reported saying when commenting on British animal feeding practices (anon 1996f). The consumption by cattle of stock feed containing material from sheep contaminated with scrapie was widely cited in media accounts as the starting point for the BSE and nvCJD story. Cattle infected with BSE may have been fed back into the stock feed chain (Collee 1997), thus creating 'cannibals'. The use of this word draws parallels with the South Fore, the Papua New Guinea tribal group, who transmitted Kuru (another type of TSE) through the consumption and handling of the brains and internal organs of dead relatives (Collee 1997).

Human consumption was mirrored, in one article, by consumption by CJD itself described as 'a degenerative disease which eats holes in [a sufferer's] brain'. It was reported widely that the common element shared by sufferers of nvCJD was beef consumption, often in the form of burgers. The importance of beefburgers as a possible source of contamination was heightened by early reports that McDonald's had effected a public relations coup by being the first hamburger chain to renounce the use British beef in its products, despite publicly stating its support for British beef (Oram 1996).

Questions about which beef products might be infectious led to construction of two categories; edible muscle was renamed as 'beef', while brains, offal and 'mechanically recovered meat' were excluded from the food chain and became 'non-beef'. Ambiguous meat products, such as 'poor-quality burgers' (Collee and Bradley 1997), sausage meat, meat pies, stock cubes, and consommés, could include spinal cord through the process of mechanically recovering meat. Regulations were not always enforced, and as a result, some banned meat products may have been allowed into the human food chain (Collee and Bradley 1997). The attention given to hamburgers or beefburgers among these doubtful products, may have been a journalistic ploy to heighten the perception of danger to children as innocent consumers. However, as steak was considered to be out of the price range of most people, hamburgers were seen as the form in which most British people ate beef, thus heightening the sense of risk to all.

One article was unusual for raising issues about the quality of burgers sold in the big chains and pointing out that although McDonald's claimed that they used 'prime beef cuts', they withdrew British beef from their products. This was linked with their poor public image and the 'McLibel' court case. McDonald's actions broadcast their patriotic allegiance but revealed yet again the contradictory forces at work, including, as one spokesman said 'Raw consumer pressures which have completely superseded science' (Oram 1996). Thus, the exclusion of meat, which McDonald's reported as safe, i.e. prime beef cuts, became a commercial necessity.

The consumption theme evolved and magnified with reports of bans on British beef in Europe and pictures of butchers shops labelling their meat to indicate it came from non-British sources. It was widely publicized that people were most likely to have contracted nvCJD from beef during 1981 to 1989 before the stricter regulations that removed material containing brains, spinal cord and other suspect material, were put in place. Consumption of British beef took on a contradictory meaning and became linked with national pride. In articles from overseas it was reported that the Queen served British beef to the French Prime Minister Chirac, and that German Chancellor Kohl chose to eat British beef instead of salmon despite supporting the beef ban in the European Union.

The emphasis on consumption in the media reinforced the link between BSE and nvCJD though it was unproven and contributed to what the Australian media themselves described as 'panic' and 'hysteria' in the British press coverage. The BSE story revealed the vulnerability of, and considerable public health concerns about, the safety of food. Reports that the 'victims' were young when they contracted nvCJD, untainted by the connotations of immorality attached to diseases like HIV/AIDS, heightened fears.

Food scares, such as BSE and nvCJD, disrupt the basic cultural classification of substances into inedible and edible and call into question the transformation of the former to the latter by the process of cooking. They may be seen in a more theoretical light, as features of a modern 'oral' society in which the individualistic body is the site of concerns over the control of what it ingests and eating itself becomes an act of 'self-fulfilment' (Falk 1994).

Consumption was often linked with 'unnatural' practices. The feeding of ruminant animal matter to ruminant animals was frequently described as unnatural in articles reporting on BSE and nvCJD[2] (Beale 1996). This theme was taken up in letters to *The Sydney Morning Herald* and *The Australian*, commenting on BSE and nvCJD, and expanded upon in articles on the food industry, making links with meat consumption in general, modern farming practices, and genetic engineering. Ripe, taking letters to the paper as evidence, suggests that it is this interpretation of BSE, that is the conversion of herbivores into carnivores and cannibals, that was most disturbing to *The Australian's* readers (Ripe 1996).

Implicit in many letters and articles was the assumption that what was unnatural was bad or dangerous. There was little discussion about how the concept of naturalness was constructed or what defined and identified the boundaries between natural and unnatural. The argument that feeding herbivores meat is unnatural (Beale 1996), is presumably based on the understanding that herbivores, in natural surroundings, do not choose to eat meat (except perhaps the placenta). Thus modern farming practices were criticized as unnatural though farming, as we know it, does not occur in nature. Cannibalism, involved in the transmission of Kuru, was also portrayed as unnatural, though its usual practitioners, tribal groups, are often represented as more natural than inhabitants of western industrial society. Nature was contrasted and set up in conflict with mankind's 'technological hubris' (Abriel 1996) which was seen to contain the seeds of its own revenge or defeat (see also Tenner 1996).

Frequently, what can be seen as unnatural in media accounts of BSE involves the transgression of boundaries. As described in press coverage, feeding ruminant meal to herbivores breached a boundary between species and resulted in a disease crossing a 'natural' boundary. A further transgression of the boundary between cattle and humans was speculated upon with the appearance of nvCJD. In the following excerpt the ease with which BSE is seen to cross between species boundaries is emphasized by the vision of prions effortlessly leaping and bounding from one species to another. However, scientific evidence suggests that the barriers between species are considerable (Collee 1997).

> If the disease could jump from one species to another, campaigners argued then surely it could leap to humans. Over the next few years, the disease (BSE) progressed by leaps and bounds. It leapt into thousands of head of cattle, and it bounded into zoo and farm and parkland creatures such as elk, mice marmosets, pigs, antelopes, kudu, oryx, eland, cheetah, puma, ocelot, domestic cat and even ostrich (Radford 1996).

Australia's natural boundaries assisted in keeping BSE from its cattle herds and, for once, the country's geographic isolation was seen as a positive force, although questions were raised about quarantine services. But for countries less isolated, the appearance of nvCJD threatened and brought into question national and international boundaries (natural or unnatural), and at both a political and symbolic level, Britain's membership of the European Union. The political and economic implications of BSE and nvCJD for the British beef industry quickly took on proportions larger than those of the original scare over the cases of nvCJD. Anxiety about national and cultural boundaries in the European Union were expressed through concerns about food, while anxiety about food and contagion focused attention on national boundaries. Within the undifferentiated European Union, countries with and without BSE could be named and, in Britain's case, isolated. The history of Europe with its dissolving and recreated boundaries, and nations consuming and being consumed by others, lends a piquancy to Britain's 'beef war' with the European Union (anon 1996g) that was heightened by the British tabloids (Arksey 1996). Thus, the story of BSE and nvCJD, raises questions about the management of other contagious diseases in the new European Union where the management of borders and boundaries is being renegotiated.

Is 'Clean, Green' Australia Victor or Victim?[3]

Separated from Europe and protected by its boundaries, Australia was situated in press coverage as potentially both victor and victim of the BSE and nvCJD crisis. Once the initial concerns about the safety of Australian beef were assuaged, the next move in press coverage was to judge the effects of the crisis on Australian beef markets. The view was expressed that Australia could benefit from the British crisis by expanding its meat markets to take up those created by bans on British beef (anon 1996). However, it was reported that Australian beef was not packaged so that it could be distinguished from British beef. Over the next month reports appeared that, in Asia as well as Europe, consumer confidence in beef in general had dwindled to the extent that Australian beef sales had dropped (Boyd 1996).

Australia and Australian beef thus became a victim of the crisis through the general fear of beef that was reported to be sweeping the world. At the same time, Australia quite explicitly attempted to benefit from the crisis in the promotion of its own beef and the image of Australia as clean and green. Australia, as the world's largest beef exporter 'is proud of its achievement in producing clean, wholesome and disease-free beef' wrote David Palmer, Manager, Food Safety and Quality Assurance, Australian Meat and Livestock Corporation in a letter to *The Sydney Morning Herald*. Quarantine laws and the 'tyranny of distance' allowed Australia to emphasize its physical and moral separation. But even in the absence of BSE, Australian beef was still contaminated by fear of the British disease. For journalists, who found it hard to maintain interest once BSE was shown to be absent in Australia, the economic contagion may well have provided the major remaining interest.

SCIENTISTS AS WHISTLE BLOWERS, SAVIOURS OR SINNERS?

Breaching natural boundaries, as in Mary Shelley's *Frankenstein* (1818) or more recently the case of transgenic pork, is perceived as a function of science. In the BSE and nvCJD story science and scientists are portrayed as saviours and whistle blowers because of their early revelations about potential dangers of BSE. They were cast in a favourable light in comparison with the British government and agencies such as MAFF that steadfastly denied any risks. However, this picture of science is framed by a larger one of distrust through the implicit and explicit linking of BSE and nvCJD with other 'unnatural' scientific and technological practices in modern farming and other domains. Such 'scientific rationalism' can accept the feeding of ruminant feed to ruminants, because as a scientist said in an newspaper interview about transgenic pork, 'once a protein is a protein it doesn't matter where it is sourced'. An article, published shortly after the BSE and nvCJD crisis commenced, reported that the Chief Scientist from BresaGen, the company that produced the 'big pig' which contains 'a bit of modified human genetic material', has a message 'DNA ... is not sacred'. 'Eating pork from BresaGen's pig ... does not mean one is eating human flesh'. Thus, in this article the 'rational scientific argument' was opposed to irrational lay fears of genetically modified food (Gilchrist 1996).

More broadly, throughout the BSE and nvCJD reporting, 'consumer confidence' was opposed to scientific rationalism by the British government, by scientists, by producers and retailers (Ellingsen 1996; Oram 1996) and by journalists themselves. Scientific endeavour was, and still is, central to the recognition, management and understanding of BSE and nvCJD and the saga raises questions about the role of scientists within government bodies and the relationship between science and the press.

Killer Proteins or Prusinic's Prions: Reporting on the science of BSE and nvCJD

During the first week of the saga in the Australian press (22 March 1996 to 27 March 1996) a number of articles, many of them from overseas sources, reported on the event from perspectives ranging from that of a public health scare, a political scandal or a major economic disaster.

In *The Sydney Morning Herald* for example, these stories framed the regular reader's perceptions of the crisis. The disease was usually described as Mad Cow Disease (rather than BSE) providing a potent image of staggering, distressed, demented cows. An adjective usually associated with humans was attached to animals; thus strengthening the sense of boundary transgression. The use of the term 'mad cow' in the press was central to its reporting on BSE as well as to the countervailing stream of jokes, funny stories and word plays on 'mad cow' that appeared in brief articles, letters and jokes.

The early articles provided little scientific explanation other than a 'possible link' between Mad Cow Disease and nvCJD. While these articles qualified the association between BSE and nvCJD as 'possible', 'probable' and as a 'link' rather than a cause, their narrative flow generally framed the link in a stronger light. For example, the first report in *The Sydney Morning Herald* on 22 March 1996, which was sourced from *Agence France-Presse*, framed the story as a combat between scientists and the government. According the article '(v)ocal scientists' had warned of the dangers for ten years and the government had 'ignored' them for political and economic purposes.

While scientists had, indeed, warned of the dangers there was still much debate within scientific circles about the link. For example, in a collection of articles in *The British Medical Journal* in late November 1995, various experts had attempted to assess the connection between BSE and nvCJD (Almond, Brown et al. 1995). European and English experts commented on biological, physiological and epidemiological studies. While few wished to deny the possibility of a risk, most were ambivalent and none claimed proof. The epidemiological studies were also unclear. One epidemiologist argued that the incidence of CJD was no higher in Britain than elsewhere in Europe, and that the increase in new cases may be due to improved diagnostic techniques. Others postulated that there was an increase of cases in the

United Kingdom. Most newspaper articles gave little hint of the uncertainty and contradiction within the body of scientific knowledge on the subject. Six months later, while there was new evidence to support the hypothesized link between BSE and nvCJD, 'there is no formal proof of the transmissibility of BSE to man' (Collee and Bradley 1997).

Descriptions of nvCJD in articles from overseas tended to highlight its more dramatic features. The headline to an article from the United States by Laurie Garrett (author of *The Coming Plague*, 1995) was 'Killer protein with no face' although the actual article was quite measured in its description of the disease (Garrett 1996). It gave a sense of the difficulties and the slow pace of research on 'prions', described as 'simply proteins' without genetic material, first isolated by Stanley Prusiner in 1982. Many articles reported on the death toll, in terms such as 'two more die' and there was frequent references to Britain 'counting the cost'.

Other articles described the 'holes' in sufferers' brains produced by a disease described as 'silent', a 'sleeper', 'always fatal', 'slow', and producing the symptoms of depression, dementia, and loss of bodily control. Such descriptions were unlikely to reduce readers' fears about nvCJD.

Articles by Australian journalists that specialized in the area of CJD and science reporting were more detailed and were balanced between being readable and presenting the scientific data on BSE and nvCJD in more critical detail than the overseas reports (see Cooke 1996; Cribb 1996). Articles by these journalists connected nvCJD with other prion diseases and discussed the wider implications of nvCJD.

Cribb's article, and one by an American journalist for *The New York Times* (Boffey 1996) were unusual because they drew attention to the 'tenuous' nature of the links between BSE and nvCJD and the danger of destroying the British beef industry based on these links.

Roving Risk—Reporting on the Unknown

One of the most problematic features of the 'science' of nvCJD was the reporting of risk, in the sense of danger (Douglas 1992). People wanted to know if they might have already contracted the disease and whether they might do so if they continued to eat British beef.

Articles in the Australian press, often from overseas, contained estimations of wildly differing numbers of people who may have contracted nvCJD. They were reported to be in the thousands, the tens of thousands, and from 'zero to millions'. Such widely varying estimations prompted a response from the editor of *The Lancet* who suggested that it would be more useful to report that scientists did not know what the risk was rather than reporting such confusing, contradictory and frightening numbers (anon 1996a).

The fearful nature of nvCJD which was emphasized in some newspaper coverage, as a new disease that was undetectable, slow and fatal, added to the concerns about the risks of contracting it. As Brunton stated 'risks of dreaded disease or serious harm, particularly when the effects of exposure are delayed or exposure is involuntary or uncontrollable, are perceived to be greater and more serious. New risks, previously unknown to science inspire particular concern and even panic' (Brunton 1996).

BSE and nvCJD were described in the typical external health risk rhetoric rather than the more familiar lifestyle risk discourse. The diseases were portrayed as risks imposed on a population which had little means of control. Many people gave up eating beef although the period of high risk had passed. Such a response may be interpreted as an attempt to take control of a situation over which individuals had no control. It has been argued that the discourse of risk is moralistic, with those at risk of the threat, in this case the consumers of beef, perceived to be 'sinned against' prompting a search for the perpetrators or 'sinners' (Douglas 1990 cited in Lupton 1993).

In other ways nvCJD offered a different risk experience from the more commonly discussed public health risks. The so-called lifestyle diseases where experts place more emphasis on the risks associated with smoking, drinking and eating 'unhealthy food' than the general population, are an example. In such cases, lay experience gives people a basis for forming their own judgements about risks (Davison, Frankel et al. 1992). With BSE and nvCJD, individuals had no personal experience upon which they could form their own risk estimations. With lifestyle diseases, experts generally warn about the risks of developing long term health problems. Individuals may use their personal bodily experience, such as putting on weight or developing a cough to assess their chances of developing a chronic health problem such as heart disease or a smoking-related disease.

In the case of BSE and nvCJD, the widely varying estimations of the risks of contracting nvCJD denied individuals an opportunity to judge their chances in comparison to the rest of the population. The 'silent' nature of nvCJD and its lengthy incubation period meant they were unable to draw upon bodily experience to assess their personal risk. One commentary drew parallels between beef eaters wondering whether they would contract nvCJD with how homosexuals felt when they heard how big AIDS had become (Tabakoff 1996). Thus, while there was no experience upon which beef eaters could draw to reduce or contextualize their risk, many may have transformed it from an objective entity as described by experts to one which they subjectively experienced (Gifford 1986).

In coverage of BSE and nvCJD, risk was seen to change depending on whether scientific experts, governments or consumers were assessing it. Over the course of the BSE and nvCJD saga, the perception of consumers' risk of contracting the disease moved from its association with very specific parts of an animal to the entire animal. It transferred from individual beasts likely to have been in contact with BSE to any cattle from Britain as newspapers reported declining beef consumption. In both European and Asian markets, beef from any country, Australia included, was perceived to be risky; falls in beef consumption were widespread. Some articles reported that the perception of the risk was attached to any red meat and, in some cases, to any meat at all. The fluid nature of risk in this case partially reflects the many unknown aspects of BSE and nvCJD, including routes of contamination and infection. As the perception of the risk spread outwards, it became more removed from the scientific assessments of the sources of risk, thus exemplifying again the disjunction between 'consumer confidence' and 'science'.

In the case of BSE and nvCJD, as in other risk discourses, the communication of risk had international political and economic implications (Lupton 1993). Germany was reported to be the country most concerned with about the risks, demanding that the ban remained on British beef until BSE was eradicated (anon 1996i). The British interpreted the German reaction to the risk of BSE and nvCJD to be as much a political, as a public health, gesture. Indeed, many of the decisions made in the management of BSE were explicitly described as being based on political and economic arguments rather than a scientific understanding.

While press reports were likely to have heightened fear of the disease, by emphasizing the high number of potential cases, and, at the same time, its unknowable nature, experts deplored the poor communication of risk (Marmot 1996), or saw it as exemplifying the need for better understanding of risk perception (Brunton 1996). Implicit in some scientific statements about the problems of risk communication was that scientific estimations of risk are the 'correct' ones and that panic over BSE and nvCJD was irrational, based on poor reporting in the media as well as general ignorance and misunderstanding of the nature and processes of science.

DISCUSSION

Science and the Press
BSE and nvCJD, like other newsworthy disease outbreaks, highlight the differences between science and the press as institutions, each with their own agenda and processes; one concerned with knowledge production based on claims of truth and the other with knowledge production that is newsworthy. One educates and the other informs.

This analysis, in common with other analyses of newspaper reporting revealed the heavy reliance on bureaucratic experts for information and commentary on BSE and nvCJD (Lupton 1995). In overseas articles these were typically the ministers of health and the ministers of agriculture, members of the SEAC committee and the scientists who had first warned of the risks of BSE to humans. Several articles in *The Sydney Morning Herald* and *The Australian* covered the story from the beef farmers' perspective emphasizing their status as victims facing economic ruin. However, just as bureaucrats and representatives of government bodies are relied upon as expert sources of information, they also tend to be identified as objects of blame, rather than business interests (Lupton 1995).

Another typical feature of newspaper reports on the diseases was their use of a body count, with references to the possibility of many more, as an attention seeking device. Headlines were used to announce the discovery of either new cases of nvCJD or deaths. While the importance and potential disaster of future fatalities associated with CJD are not to be denied, the number of deaths from nvCJD at present is small in comparison to diseases such malaria or road fatalities. This emphasis on the body count was confused in the British press, by not distinguishing between nvCJD and sporadic CJD which was discovered many years ago. Four farm workers that were cited as nvCJD cases were actually cases of sporadic CJD. Although this did not alter the numbers of cases, it confused speculation on the modes of transmission.

The physical and moral distance from the outbreak of BSE allowed Australian journalists to take a more distanced, less passionate, and less 'hysterical' view of the crisis than British counterparts.

The interspersing of local and overseas articles was a technique through which readers were alternatively alarmed and reassured. Overseas articles raised concerns about the frightening nature of CJD and its potential disasters while local articles reassured readers that there was no danger of transmission from BSE here. The commentary style of local articles framed the BSE and nvCJD saga in a broader and less risky perspective. This pattern of reporting, which de-emphasizes local catastrophes and exaggerates the unpleasant and dangerous consequences of events elsewhere, appears to be a general feature of press coverage (Spencer and Triche 1994).

The press coverage provided little detail about the diseases at the centre of the story. With the exception of articles written by expert journalists, the technical explanations of BSE and nvCJD in most articles were restricted to one or two sentences. The complexity and mystery of BSE and nvCJD may have been daunting for journalists who had no training or experience in the area of science or medical reporting.

A central difficulty for journalists in reporting on BSE and nvCJD research and in determining its scientific validity, was that very little science had been done on the subject. Scientific bodies stated that 'further data are urgently required' (The WHO consultation (14 to 16 May 1996) cited in BSE/nvCJD Scientific Advisory Group, 1996). The intense media, public and political interest occurred at a time when there was a lack of scientific evidence on all aspects of BSE and nvCJD. Even the identification of nvCJD as a new and distinct type of CJD in humans was uncertain with concern that these cases may have been found because of better surveillance. Questions about of the link between BSE and nvCJD, the mode of transmission of BSE between cows, and to humans, were unanswered along with many others including the management of BSE in British herds (Butler 1996).

BSE and nvCJD thus exemplified one of the major difficulties in the press coverage of science. When a crisis such as this occurs, the press, and others, expect answers even though research findings have not been available in the scientific community long enough to be adequately discussed. A French epidemiologist commenting on the saga described how in science, the publication of new findings initiates scientific discussion and interpretation rather than concluding them. This scientific process is not only a problem for the media who are anxious to report new findings as soon as they are available. It also becomes important, as in the case of BSE and nvCJD, when the science concerns public health issues where governments must make policy decisions while the science is in its infancy. At the time the BSE and nvCJD story broke in 1996 scientists were unable to answer definitively many of the questions that the British government and the general population were asking about BSE and nvCJD.

The reporting on BSE and nvCJD in Australia conformed with existing analyses of the different agendas of the media and science, such as the media's need to produce newsworthy copy informing the public about what is interesting and topical (Goodall 1987). They work under constraints of time and space (Klaidman 1990). Technology, notably computers and satellites has speeded up communication enormously allowing newspapers to transmit stories world-wide within hours. In contrast, while technology has sped up the process of science, it has enabled scientists to increase the complexity and specialization of their knowledge production.

CJD as an Epidemic of the Late Twentieth Century

nvCJD was described as an epidemic in press coverage. It conforms to technical definitions of an epidemic because it was the 'first invasion of a disease not previously recognized [which] may be sufficient evidence to be considered an epidemic' (Last 1995:54). As well as having a technical definition, the use of the word 'epidemic' is highly emotional, linked in many people's minds with fear and sudden, mysterious, widespread death (Rosenberg 1992; Lupton 1995). It is associated with traditional plagues like the Black Death and the more recently discovered diseases, like Ebola, outbreaks of which have received widespread publicity. Descriptions of nvCJD in the press draw upon both uses of the word to raise fears about it.

BSE and nvCJD were sometimes also compared to HIV/AIDs. Without sophisticated laboratory techniques nvCJD, like HIV/AIDs, would not have been known as a distinct disease or as an epidemic (Rosenberg 1992:290). Indeed, in earlier times sporadic CJD was seen as one of many forms of dementia. Thus the crucial role of the scientist in the recognition and understanding of the disease forces science and the press into an uneasy alliance. Typical also of other epidemics of this historic period is the complexity of the local, state and international institutions that must respond to it (Rosenberg 1992:290). In the case of nvCJD, its links with BSE demanded a coordinated response from the agricultural, veterinary, health and economic experts at all levels as well as trade experts in the international arena. Instead, BSE and nvCJD provoked conflict between these institutions with each attempting to represent their own constituencies.

Drawing it all together is the media. Such an epidemic is a 'media reality' in that most people only experience the epidemic and make sense of it through media reports (Rosenberg 1992:290). The media makes it possible for a disease like nvCJD to become international, experienced in Australia, Japan and Russia. The complexity of BSE and nvCJD is magnified by media which contribute to the multiple frames of meaning that can be placed on such diseases, as they make it relevant to countries around the world.

The Epidemic as a Moral Tale

Epidemics can be seen as events which are understood within social and moral frameworks. Traditionally, they were believed to be divine retribution for individual and community sins. Over the centuries such spiritual explanations have made room for more rationalistic ones (Rosenberg 1992:288). And though current rational explanations of BSE and nvCJD favour the prion, press coverage reveals another tale. Its narrative structure follows that of older epidemics. After the initial reluctance to acknowledge an epidemic comes acceptance of its existence, followed by fear, panic and blame. Community rituals of propitiation are made (Rosenberg 1992:279) which, in this case were media visions of burning cow carcasses.

Within this structure, a moral tale (Lupton 1995) can be seen to unfold. It was one of humans, motivated by greed and self-interest, tampering with nature and transgressing boundaries by feeding unnatural foods to animals. Blame was attributed to the Conservatives, the Thatcher government, John Major, MAFF and big business in general. As the story progressed the consequences of these sins were revealed with the appearance of BSE and nvCJD which mirrored the first half of the story by leaping species and national boundaries. The resulting punishment of illness and death was magnified by the subsequent destruction of Britain's beef industry, the beef bans by the European Union and Britain's isolation and international humiliation. The narrative structure of articles throughout the period until the end of June told this story starting with discovery of the disease, the linking with feeding practices, and revelations that the government deregulated the industry and ignored the warnings of science. The later articles focus on the disaster that followed.

Meanwhile this moral tale also revealed the multiple frames of meaning (Rosenberg 1992:288) that can be placed on the BSE and nvCJD saga. The complex history and involvement of many diverse subject areas in the BSE and nvCJD story makes it a malleable and adaptable tale, lending itself to many causes. It was used to raise questions about food safety in Australia and the modern technological management of food production, distribution and storage. Vegetarians drew conclusions about the dangers of meat and meat eaters questioned farming practices. Experts drew upon BSE and nvCJD to exemplify their arguments and draw lessons from the experience (Jopson 1996; McMichael 1996). Scientists also employed BSE and nvCJD to draw attention to the dangers of reduced funding and the reliance on government agencies, such as MAFF, rather than independent research (Gready 1996). Individuals wrote letters to newspapers commenting on the meaning of BSE and nvCJD for a range of issues.

CONCLUSION

The BSE and nvCJD saga draws upon ancient fears of transgressing boundaries and upsetting the natural order. As in earlier epidemics moral concepts of risk and blame are involved. But, typical of a late twentieth century epidemic, it has had multiple frames of meaning and interpretation placed upon it. Among these is the oft-repeated message of the importance of consumer confidence in the safety of their food, which was contrasted to the rationality of scientific statements of risks. Thus, public distrust in the institutions of government and science was exposed. The saga reveals again the crucial role played by the media in the maintenance or destruction of trust because they 'help to create the unarticulated assumptions and fundamental beliefs that underlie personal decisions, public policies, and clinical practices.' (Nelkin 1996).

ACKNOWLEDGEMENTS

The authors acknowledge the valuable contributions of the following people: Emily Mauldon, who conducted a literature search and compiled much of the textual data; Stephen Fitzpatrick, who also obtained material for us; and Tony Adams, Jennifer Cooke, and Julian Cribb who made insightful comments on the subject.

NOTES

[1] Even this is in contention. Some farmers claim that there have always been cases of cows with the 'staggers'—one of the symptoms of BSE.

[2] Professor Peter Singer at Monash University's Centre for Human Bioethics, and others were cited using this argument.

[3] This term has been used in several articles. See, for example Cribb 1996a.

REFERENCES

Abriel, V. (1996). A bitter pill to swallow. The Australian, April 15: 13.

Almond, J. W., Brown, P. et al. (1995). 'Creutzfeldt-Jakob Disease and Bovine Spongiform Encephalopathy: Any connection?' British Medical Journal, **311**: 1415-1421.

anon (1996). Lessons in mad cow calamity. The Australian, March 27: 8.

anon (1996a). Editorial: Betraying the public over nvCJD risk. The Lancet, **348**: 1529.

anon (1996b). Editorial: Less beef, more brain. The Lancet, **347**: 915.

anon (1996c). The cattle plague. The Australian, March 27: 13.

anon (1996d). Thatcher cabinet 'hid' mad cow risk, says MP. The Sydney Morning Herald, March 25: 8.

anon (1996e). Steps to an awful discovery. The Weekend Australian, March 30-31: 26.

anon (1996f). Major erupts as Europe confirms world beef ban. The Sydney Morning Herald, March 29: 10.

anon (1996g). British beef. The Australian, May 31: 10.

anon (1996h). Bovril safe. The Sydney Morning Herald, March 26: 4.

anon (1996i). Britain agrees to mad-cow slaughter. The Sydney Morning Herald, April 4: 1.

Arksey, N. (1996). I'll steak my life on it, guv. The Australian, May 30: 13.

Beale, B. (1996). Mad cow scare leads to new feed rules. The Sydney Morning Herald, May 8: 1.

Boffey, P. (1996). Even today, jury is out on the cause. The Sydney Morning Herald, March 30: 17.

Boyd, T. (1996). Mad cow fears hit Asia. The Australian Financial Review, May 31: 23.

Brunton, C. (1996). 'Barmy beef, brain eating bugs, bad blood and the problems of risk communication.' Snow's Field: The Newsletter of the Australasian Faculty of Public Health Medicine **6**(2): 1-2.

BSE/CJD Scientific Advisory Group (1996). Report to the interdepartmental advisory task force on BSE and CJD. Canberra.

Butler, D. (1996). 'Mad cow politics tries to corral science'. Nature **383**: 209.

Collee, J. G. (1997). BSE: A decade on, part 1. The Lancet **349**: 636-41.

Collee, J. G., Bradley, R. (1997). 'BSE: A decade on, part 2'. The Lancet **349**: 715-721.

Cooke, J. (1996). Burning questions. The Sydney Morning Herald, March 29: 13.

Cribb, J. (1996). The 'sleeper' nightmare. The Weekend Australian, March 30-31: 27.

Cribb, J. (1996a). Bizarre disease difficult to expose. The Australian, March 27: 13.

Davison, C., Frankel, S. et al. (1992). 'The limits of lifestyle: Reassessing "fatalism" in the popular culture of illness prevention'. Social Science and Medicine **34**(6): 675-685.

Douglas, M. (1992). Risk and Blame: Essays in cultural theory. London, Routledge.

Ellingsen, P. (1996). Death and devastation down on the farm. The Sydney Morning Herald, March 30: 33.

Ellingsen, P. (1996). Major in European Union fury as two more die. The Sydney Morning Herald, March 27: 9.

Falk, P. (1994). The Consuming Body. London, Sage.

Garrett, L. (1995). The Coming Plague: Newly emerging diseases in a world out of balance. New York, Farrar, Strauss and Giroux.

Garrett, L. (1996). Killer protein with no face: The prion mystery beef crisis: Britain counts the cost. The Sydney Morning Herald, March 27: 9.

Gifford, S. M. (1986). The meaning of lumps: A case study of the ambiguities of risk. Anthropology and Epidemiology. C. R. Janes, R. Stall and S. M. Gifford, D. Reidel Publishing Company.

Gilchrist, G. (1996). Future food: Is it so hard to swallow? Gene Cuisine. The Sydney Morning Herald, March 27: 11.

Goodall, R. (1987). Role of mass media in scientific controversy. Scientific Controversies. H. T. Engelhardt and A. L. Caplan, Cambridge, Cambridge University Press.

Gready, J. (1996). 'Mad-cow Disease and UK government research policy: What went wrong.' Australian Society for Biochemistry and Molecular Biology Inc **27**(5): 3-5.

Hoy, A. , Cooke, J. (1996). Mad Cow Disease: Even chocolate is suspect now. The Sydney Morning Herald, March 23: 3.

Jopson, D. (1996). How civilisation is killing us. The Sydney Morning Herald, April 4: 11.

Klaidman, S. (1990). 'How well the media report health risk'. Daedalus **119**(4): 119-132.

Last, J. M., Ed. (1995). A Dictionary of Epidemiology. Oxford, Oxford University Press.

Lupton, D. (1993). 'Risk as moral danger: The social and political functions of risk discourse in public health'. International Journal of Health Services **23**(3): 425-435.

Lupton, D. (1995). 'Anatomy of an epidemic'. Media Information Australia **76**: 92-99.

Marmot, M. (1996). 'Editorial: From alcohol and breast cancer to beef and BSE—improving our communication of risk'. American Journal of Public Health **86**(7): 921-922.

McMichael, A. J. (1996). 'Bovine spongiform encephalopathy: Its wider meaning for population health'. British Medical Journal **312**: 1313-1314.

Nelkin, D. (1996). 'An uneasy relationship: The tensions between medicine and the media'. The Lancet **347**: 1600-1603.

Oram, R. (1996). Consumers dictate terms on burgers. The Australian, March 27: 13.

Parkinson, T. (1995). Mad Cow Disease: A scandal of dither and delay. The Weekend Australian, March 30-31: 26-27.

Radford, T. (1996). Deadly cattle epidemic keeps scientists puzzled. The Sydney Morning Herald, March 23: 15.

Ripe, C. (1996). Negligence feeds beef contamination. The Weekend Australian, April 20: Review 4.

Rosenberg, C. E. (1992). Explaining Epidemics and Other Studies in the History of Medicine. Cambridge, Cambridge University Press.

Spencer, W., Triche, E. (1994). 'Media construction of risk and safety: Differential framings of hazard events'. Sociological Inquiry 64(2): 199-213.

Stott, D. (1996). Five UK beef food products banned. The Sydney Morning Herald, March 30: 5.

Tabakoff, J. (1996). Lots at steak. The Sydney Morning Herald, March 30: 2.

Tenner, E. (1996). Why Things Bite Back. London, Fourth Estate.

Will, R., Ironside, J. et al. (1996). 'A new variant of Creutzfeldt-Jakob disease in the UK'. The Lancet 347: 921-925.

Woolford, D. (1996). Agribusiness deadly triangle blamed for 'the disaster waiting to happen'. The Sydney Morning Herald, March 30: 17.

HOW NOW MAD COW?
Michael Fitzpatrick

In October 1996 seven months after the take-off of the great mad cow panic in Britain, the first hard evidence was published of a link between BSE and nvCJD reported in ten young people earlier in the year. The team headed by Professor John Collinge at Saint Mary's Hospital in London identified a distinctive molecular 'signature' which not only distinguished nvCJD from its familiar forms, but could also be found in BSE itself and in cases of disease in other animal species (mice, cats, macaque monkeys) resulting from experimental exposure to BSE (Collinge et al. October 1996). This elegant piece of research, though not conclusive, provided the first scientific backing for what was previously conjecture.

In the spring of 1996, I wrote a series of articles challenging the irrationality of the mad cow panic, commenting that this was a health scare 'not about a disease, but about the possibility of a disease' and emphasizing that the supposed link between BSE and CJD remained unsubstantiated (Fitzpatrick, February 1996, May 1996). In a letter published in the *British Medical Journal* I particularly emphasized the role of scientists in promoting the scare (April 1996). Did this new research now offer retrospective justification for the mad cow panic? Should we now exonerate the British government and its scientific advisers?

The critical consensus that emerged in the course of the year was that up to 20 March, when government ministers first acknowledged the possibility of a link between BSE and CJD, the politicians and the scientists were guilty of at least prevarication and cover-up, if not of incompetence and undue influence from the farming lobby. Though commentators may disagree about the government's subsequent handling of the diverse consequences of the panic, they broadly welcomed its decision to publicize concerns about the risks of BSE, after nearly a decade of playing down fears of a link with CJD.

I take a different view. It seems to me that, until March, both the scientists and the government handled the BSE problem appropriately. It was their collective loss of nerve in March that triggered the panic, which was duly amplified by the media and spread rapidly among a public that is highly susceptible to scares about health and environmental issues.

THE MARCH DEBACLE

In his statement to the House of Commons on 20 March, Health Secretary Stephen Dorrell quoted from the document he had received from the government's SEAC. This committee had considered reports of ten cases of CJD among people under the age of forty-two received by the specialist surveillance unit in Edinburgh and had come to the following conclusion:

> On current data and in the absence of any credible alternative, the most likely explanation at present is that these cases are linked to exposure to BSE before the introduction of the specified bovine offal ban in 1989 (*The Times*, 21 March 1996).

Dorrell emphasized that there was 'no scientific evidence that BSE can be transmitted to man by beef', and drew attention to the committee's conviction that 'the risk from eating beef is now likely to be extremely small'. However, recognizing that 'parents will be concerned about the implications for their children', he announced that he had requested that the committee provide specific advice on this question following its next meeting.

Apart from drawing attention to the possible link between BSE and the new cases of CJD, there was little further of substance either in Dorrell's statement, or that from Agriculture Minister Douglas Hogg. Nor indeed did the statement issued by Chief Medical Officer Sir Kenneth Calman, and immediately sent by fax to every doctor in the country, add much. The government's senior officers emphasized that measures already in place to control BSE should be rigorously enforced and they declared a commitment to further research. The only specific measures introduced were the ruling that cattle over the age of thirty months should be deboned in specified plants, to prevent the 'extremely small risk of transmission from non-muscle parts of the carcass', and a ban on use of mammalian meat and bonemeal in feed for all farm animals. These regulations amounted to a minor tightening up of procedures introduced in 1988 to 1989 in response to the first recognition of the BSE epidemic.

The immediate effect of the fear of Mad Cow Disease spreading to humans was a spate of headlines like that in the next day's *Daily Mirror*—MAD COW CAN KILL—and a dramatic fall in the consumption of beef. The Vegetarian Society estimated later in the year that around one million people in Britain immediately gave up eating beef. In response to the climate of fear about beef, schools, hospitals and other institutions were obliged to remove it from their menus. When McDonald's announced an end to the use of British beef in its burgers, other fast food chains followed suit.

Supermarkets, butchers and wholesalers reported a slump in sales: six months later they remained 15% below the normal level.

Within days the European Union and other overseas importers banned British beef, though this was not enough to prevent a sharp fall in demand for supposedly BSE-free continental beef. In the ensuing months the British government engaged in increasingly acrimonious disputes with its European Union partners over the extent of the mass slaughter of British cattle required to assuage continental fears of contamination.

The impact on the British meat industry—worth four billion pounds a year—was catastrophic. Britain has more than forty thousand dairy farmers and ninety-five thousand in beef; around half of all British farmers derive all or part of their income from beef. Some thirty thousand more work in slaughtering, processing and transportation. Early estimates suggested an increase of the trade gap of up to one and a half billion pounds as a result of the European Union ban. In April, a spokesman for the Transport and General Workers Union told a parliamentary inquiry that eight thousand people had been laid off or made redundant as a result of the scare. As stories began to reach the press about farmers committing suicide, the government announced a package of compensation worth five hundred and fifty million pounds. Twelve months later the estimated cost of the mass slaughter policy passed three billion pounds.

Every case of CJD, once a rare and obscure condition, now attracted national publicity. In April, Edinburgh neurologist Professor Peter Behan revealed to the media the case of a fifteen year-old girl whom he believed had acquired CJD from eating a beefburger

(*The Times*, 30 April). In August, Durham coroner Geoffrey Burt recommended a verdict of death 'by misadventure' (instead of the customary 'natural causes') on a man who had died from CJD. He concluded that 'on the balance of probabilities', death had resulted from eating 'something like a beefburger infected with BSE' (*The Times*, 20 August). In October, a coroner in Belfast ruled that a thirty-year old engineer had died from CJD, 'probably' transmitted from BSE (*The Times*, 29 October). The notion of CJD as 'the human form of Mad Cow Disease' became firmly established in the national consciousness.

Though the scare about BSE and CJD had serious economic and social consequences, there were some who thought that it was long overdue. Since the late 1980s a small group of medical authorities—notably consultant microbiologist Professor Richard Lacey and his protege Dr Stephen Dealler—had repeatedly criticized what they regarded as the complacency of the authorities over the risks of BSE. They alleged that the farming lobby exerted undue influence on MAFF, and that MAFF in turn swayed other government ministries and the scientists. They could not prove a link between BSE and CJD, but their point was that if it turned out that transmission were possible, a catastrophic human epidemic could result. The developments of 1996 appeared to vindicate the critics and they were certainly quick to seize the limelight. But were they right?

THE SPECTRE OF BSE

The spectre of BSE spreading to humans in the form of CJD was first raised publicly in a brief article in the *British Medical Journal* in June 1988 (Holt and Phillips 1988). This article, by a dietitian and a junior hospital doctor, challenged what they characterized as the 'alarming indifference' of the medical profession and the public to the risks of BSE, which had first been recognized less than two years earlier. The authors drew attention to the use of brain-derived products in the British food industry, the lack of strict regulation of meat processing and the availability of raw brain and spinal cord tissues. They concluded ominously that 'if transmission has already occurred to man it might be years before infected individuals succumb'.

This article provoked a briskly dismissive response from Baker and Ridley, two leading British authorities in the field of TSEs, who described it as 'unnecessarily alarmist' (Baker and Ridley 1988):

> There is no evidence, however, that CJD results from eating tissue infected with scrapie, even though scrapie is common in British sheep. There is, therefore, little reason to believe that BSE will present any greater threat to humans than scrapie.

This statement brought the debate to an abrupt end. It remained the consensus among the experts in the field up to the March 1996 debacle.

The scientists did not, however, rule out the possibility of BSE being transmissible. Though the report of the committee of inquiry chaired by Oxford zoology professor Richard Southwood, published in February 1989, was generally reassuring, it acknowledged that transmission could occur and recommended measures of surveillance and control (Southwood 1989). The report pointed out the long incubation period of spongiform encephalopathies in humans and emphasized the importance of specialist scrutiny of cases 'so that they can report on any atypical cases or changing patterns in the incidence of the disease'. As a result the Edinburgh surveillance unit was established the following year.

The Southwood report also made specific policy recommendations:

> Concerned at the remote chance that this new infection could be transmitted orally to man, we recommend the destruction of carcases of cattle with suspected BSE and prohibition of the use of milk from such cows for humans.

These measures, together with a ban on the use of 'meat and bone meal' feeds (which had rapidly been identified as the common feature of the early outbreaks), were in fact implemented in 1988 before the report was published. The Southwood report also led to the establishment of SEAC whose first report in June 1989 recommended a ban on 'specified bovine offals'. This was implemented, despite some opposition from MAFF and the farmers, in November 1989. This ban prohibited the use of brain, spinal cord, spleen, tonsils and thymus from any cattle over six months of age.

Thus within three years of the first case of BSE appearing, the scientists had identified the likely cause and the government had introduced measures to prevent it from passing into the human food chain. Furthermore, it had established a system of expert surveillance as well as sponsoring further research into different aspects of the problem.

No doubt the scientists could have produced results even more quickly; no doubt the government could have acted even more promptly to curtail the spread of BSE and the processing of infected beef; no doubt too the new regulations in the abbatoirs could have been enforced more stringently. But these are criticisms that can be made of any official policy and are easily made in retrospect;

they have no particular salience in relation to the mad cow crisis. This point is well made by J. Ralph Blanchfield of the Institute of Food Science and Technology, an authoritative commentator on the BSE crisis:

> Although one may criticize aspects of the United Kingdom government's speed of introduction of some measures and the earlier failure in some instances to enforce legally-established measures stringently enough, it should be appreciated that all the measures relating to the human food chain, from the 1989 specified offals ban onwards, were on the 'as if' or precautionary principle, i.e. as if transmission to humans could occur (Blanchfield 1996).

In response to periodic flutters of public anxiety about BSE—notably when reports appeared of it spreading to cats in 1990—the authorities simply reiterated the line that as there was no evidence of any risk to human beings, beef should be considered safe. In all the circumstances, this was a reasonable position. In May 1990, Agriculture Minister, John Selwyn Gummer's attempt to reassure the public, by stuffing a beefburger into his daughter's mouth, notoriously backfired because of her refusal to eat it. But at least it showed his confidence in British beef.

The biggest challenge to the official line came in late 1995 when the eminent neuropathologist Sir Bernard Tomlinson told a radio interviewer that he had given up eating beef because of his fear of BSE. As other authorities lined up on either side of the debate, schools and other institutions took beef off the menu and pre-Christmas beef sales slumped. However, the end of the year figures showed a decline in cases of CJD (from fifty-nine in 1994 to forty-five in 1995) and there was nothing to suggest either that recent cases of CJD were in any way unusual or in any way linked to exposure to BSE-infected beef. The line held.

THE PROPHETS OF DOOM

The most persistent critic of government policy on the BSE epidemic is the Leeds-based microbiologist Richard Lacey (Lacey 1991, 1994). Indeed he has also challenged official policy on salmonella, E Coli and other infectious diseases. He does not claim to have demonstrated a link between BSE and CJD, but he does insist that the risk of transmission is much greater than has been acknowledged and that more drastic measures (notably the slaughter of more cattle) are necessary to deal with it. Upholders of the mainstream position have accused Lacey of basing his argument on three misconceptions.

They point out that he exaggerates the role of infection and underestimates the role of genetics in the pathogenesis of the TSEs. Thus though some 15% of cases of CJD are familial, there is now known to be a substantial genetic contribution to sporadic cases. However, Lacey implies that CJD must always have been caught from somewhere—specifically from cattle in which BSE has not yet been diagnosed. But this cannot explain the stable incidence of CJD worldwide, including Australia where the sheep have no scrapie and even among Hindus in India, who do not eat beef.

Lacey assumes the vertical transmission of BSE, from cow to calf (through prenatal or perinatal transplacental transfer of an infective agent, or through some other mechanism associated with birth or feeding). For Lacey this explains the persistence of the bovine epidemic, in particular of the phenomenon of infected cattle 'born after the ban' on infected feeds, and raises the spectre of BSE becoming endemic, unless virtually the entire national herd is eradicated. In an authoritative survey, Ridley and Baker conclude that 'the probability of maternal transmission of spongiform encephalopathy in any species should be viewed with the greatest scepticism' (Ridley and Baker October 1995). A large scale epidemiological study published in 1995 failed to reveal evidence of vertical transmisssion of BSE (Hoinville et al. 1995).

Lacey also assumes that the proportion of animal species into which BSE can be transmitted experimentally can be translated into an approximation of the risk to humans. Thus, in an article written jointly with Dealler, he points out that 'about 50% of species can be infected from any one species with an encephalopathy' (Dealler and Lacey 1991). As Collee replied in the same issue, this statement 'is not meaningful unless the transmission rate is related to the range of species and the challenge routes used' (Collee 1991). On these rather insubstantial foundations, Lacey has challenged the official position, demanding drastic measures of 'quarantine, cessation of breeding, slaughter and replenishment' to control BSE (Lacey 1996).

Stephen Dealler, formerly Lacey's junior in Leeds, but now himself a consultant in Burnley, Lancashire, has taken up his cause. His hurriedly-published personal account, *Lethal Legacy: BSE—the search for the truth* offers a rather bizarre account that is more revealing of its author than it of the BSE crisis (Dealler 1996). The book is written in the style of a script for the X-Files in which the intrepid author seeks the truth against forces of darkness which not only try to frustrate his inquiries and prevent publication of his investigations, but are also responsible for the mysterious disappearance of his computer discs. But Dealler is not alone! At several points in his text he records the arrival of anonymous letters on unheaded notepaper—'postmark illegible'—encouraging him against despondency and urging him on to further heroic exploits.

Dealler is not inhibited by the lack of evidence for a link between BSE and CJD. Indeed for him the link has the character of an article of faith, an assumption which does not require proof. He has taken over from Lacey the argument that the proportion of animal species to which BSE can be transmitted can be directly translated into an estimate of the risk of transmission to humans: this risk supposedly increased from 50% in 1991 to 70% in 1996. Dealler combines this inflation of risk with the precautionary principle: humans must be assumed to be at risk until they are shown not to be (Dealler 1996, p. 36). According to this logic, everybody should stop eating beef and the beef trade should be liquidated, and perhaps in ten years time we will know whether this was justified or not. Of course, we may never know, but you can't be too careful!

Dealler's major personal contribution to the mad cow controversy is his calculation of the quantity of beef infected with BSE that has entered the human food chain and of the risks of transmission of BSE by different sized doses of infected particles. Quite apart from the difficulties in quantifying the BSE-infected tissue, these calculations assume the possibility of transmission by the oral route. The results, published in Dealler's extensive statistical appendices, confirm that the numbers of people in the United Kingdom who would be expected to have eaten more than an indicated potentially infective dose by 1997, vary according to different variables, between zero and thirty-four and a quarter million (Dealler 1996, p. 282). In other words, even if BSE can cause CJD it is possible, according to Dealler's model, either that nobody will get it or that virtually the entire population will be wiped out. Perhaps if Dealler had consulted a few farmers instead of his computer spread sheets he might have gained some insights into the usefulness of such calculations.

Another critical account of the government's handling of BSE, by Brian Ford of the Institute of Biology, was published before Collinge's definitive demonstration of a BSE-CJD link. It reveals why the critics were happy to assume that 'the sensible conclusion at this stage' (that is, before there was any evidence for this conclusion) was that the cases of nvCJD were the result of the transmission of BSE to humans:

> It is sensible because it heightens official concern, and will encourage the government to take a long-term view of the problem. If it helps the eradication of BSE ... it can only be for the good. However, there is still no scientific reason to suppose that these new cases arose from infected beef (Ford 1996, p. 158).

In other words the facts—scientific evidence of the link between BSE and CJD—are of secondary importance to the conviction that it is necessary to heighten official (and inevitably also popular) concern about BSE.

Ford's argument is analogous to that of supporters of the AIDS scare who now freely concede that the government exaggerated the risks of heterosexual spread, but insist that this was 'a good lie' because it encouraged more restraint in sexual behaviour (Lawson 1996). The cynicism underlying the mad cow panic—and indeed of similar health scares—is revealed: facts are shamelessly marshalled in the service of propaganda.

It is perhaps not surprising, given the feebleness of their critique, that the promoters of the mad cow scare made little headway before 1996. Contributors to a symposium on the question 'CJD and BSE: Any connection?' in the *British Medical Journal* in November 1995, gave an overwhelmingly negative answer (Almond 1995). Though everybody emphasized the importance of continuing research and surveillance—and the impossibility of categorical reassurance—the consensus was that the investigation of recent cases did not reveal any connection. The only discordant note was struck by the Cambridge statistician Sheila Gore who concluded that a number of recent cases of CJD in farmers and young adults were 'more than happenstance' and signalled 'an epidemiological alert' (Gore 1995). Contributors from the Netherlands summed up the prevailing view: 'taken together, the epidemiological evidence does not point to a causal link between BSE and CJD' (Hofman and Wientjens 1995).

The publication in December of the results of early experiments on transgenic mice at Collinge's lab at Saint Mary's, suggesting that the agent responsible for BSE could not cross the 'species barrier' into humans, gave an end of year boost to the confidence of the supporters of the mainstream view (Collinge December 1995).

WHO'S MAD?

Then, a mere three months later, everything fell apart. On 8 March the Edinburgh Surveillance Unit informed SEAC that it had identified ten cases of what was to become known as nvCJD. They were much younger than typical cases (all under forty-two), they tended to present with behavioural and psychiatric disturbances and a staggering gait before developing the typical rapidly progressive dementia. Microscopic examination of biopsy or post-mortem specimens of brain tissues revealed a distinctive and consistent pathological pattern. Furthermore, none of these patients had recognized risk factors, such as a history of neurosurgical procedures or treatment with human growth hormone, or the distinctive genetic marker that tends to predispose to CJD.

Though there was still no evidence of a link between the new cases and BSE, this was understandably the first thought of everybody involved. It appeared that, after years of maintaining that human transmission was unlikely to happen, the scientists on SEAC were confronted with the possibility that the nightmare scenario predicted by Lacey and Dealler might be beginning to unfold. They immediately advised the government about the identification of nvCJD and of their view that 'the most likely' explanation was transmission from BSE. In fact, this could only be considered the most likely explanation in the absence of any more convincing alternative. Given the high level of uncertainty about many aspects of BSE and CJD, further research and monitoring of developments were the key requirements.

In fact, instead of discreetly endorsing the good work of the scientists and keeping a watchful eye on developments, government ministers chose to make a major public issue out of what was in essence a matter of concern to the departments of agriculture and health. It seemed that the scientists, rattled by the appearance of nvCJD in defiance of their expectations, had communicated their anxieties to the politicians. The politicians, in turn, transmitted their anxieties to the public in such a way that panic was inevitable.

Being advised that you face only a small risk of a devastating neurodegenerative disorder, one that is untreatable and progresses rapidly to dementia and death, is scarcely reassuring, particularly when you had previously been told repeatedly that you faced no risk at all. Any confession of uncertainty in relation to children in these circumstances could only be regarded as highly alarming, especially as the distinctive feature of the new cases was their early age of onset (at least two cases had been reported in teenagers and had already received publicity). If Dorrell had planned to provoke alarm it is difficult to imagine how he could have gone about it better. The refusal of both Dorrell and Hogg to recommend beef to their own children—in pointed contrast to Gummer's bold gesture in 1990—revealed the ministers' lack of confidence and further exacerbated public fears.

The central question is—given that measures had been in place to keep BSE out of the human food chain for more than six years, why was it necessary to give such major publicity to the emergence of nvCJD, an exotic variant of a rare disease? The announcement had no public health value: if people had been exposed to the danger of BSE transmission, this must have been before the 1989 offal ban and there was nothing further that anybody could do to avoid BSE. The additional regulations on abbatoir procedure were more a token display of rigour than of real practical importance. The government was not providing any useful information, only an invitation to panic about a risk that was indeterminate and still possibly non-existent.

The media, already sensitized to public anxieties about Mad Cow Disease in the earlier minor scares, seized on the dramatic about turn in the official line. Given that the details of the cases of nvCJD had yet to be published (they finally appeared in *The Lancet* a fortnight later—see Will et al. 1996), journalists had to rely on the politicians and the experts for information. While Lacey and Dealler were available as ever to expound the latest version of their doomsday scenario, the novel feature of the March panic was that the views of some of the mainstream authorities now appeared little different.

While Sir Kenneth Calman, the government's chief medical officer, was defiantly declaring that he would carry on eating beef, SEAC chair Professor John Pattison conceded that he would not feed it to his grandchildren. Whereas Lacey had attracted condemnation for his statement in 1990 that BSE was 'much more serious than AIDS', now Pattison conceded that 'an epidemic on the scale of AIDS was possible'. Members of SEAC now speculated wildly in the press about the possibility of the death rate from CJD reaching up to one hundred thousand (Dr Mike Painter) or even as high as five hundred thousand (Professor Pattison). In this overheated climate, even Dealler's doomsday toll of thirty-four million could begin to seem possible.

The atmosphere of panic was as much evident in sober medical journals as in the tabloid press. In a remarkable editorial in the *British Medical Journal* at the end of March, the American authority Paul Brown recalled his comment in the November symposium that the available evidence suggested 'a negligible risk to humans', only to confess that 'it now appears that I was wrong' (Brown 1995, 1996). However, he adduced no new evidence to justify this about turn, simply repeating the now familiar refrain that that 'no better explanation is presently forthcoming'. As I wrote in reply, 'being unable to advance a better explanation than that offered by a hypothesis for which there is only the weakest circumstantial backing is a dubious basis for endorsing that hypothesis' (Fitzpatrick April 1996). Yet within a few sentences, Brown was raising the spectre of a 'potential medical catastrophe'. My comment was that 'if an eminent scientist can swing in four months from characterizing BSE as a negligible risk to warning of potential catastrophe, is it any wonder that the public is confused and frightened?'

It is worth recalling the final point in Brown's contribution to the November symposium:

> There does not seem to be any need for new governmental hearings, committee meetings, or parliamentary debates about what more might be done because the precautions were taken some years ago to eliminate potentially infectious products from commercial distribution were both logical and thorough (Brown 1995).

This was as true in March as it had been four months earlier. Yet instead of urging the scientists to calm down and carry on with their work, ministers launched into precisely the sort of high profile treatment of BSE/CJD that Brown had emphasized was unnecessary—though now with his approval.

In a second *British Medical Journal* editorial on the same subject, Sheila Gore—who had challenged the consensus against the BSE/CJD link in the November symposium—now deployed fervid metaphors about British beef consumers continuing 'to play Russian roulette' (Gore 1995, 1996). With rhetorical flourish she demanded 'let us have done with misleading the profession, the public and the press', and insisted that 'all evidence must be quantified'. But as there was then no evidence for a link between BSE and CJD, it could not be quantified. However, applying the Russian roulette model to quantify the risks of eating beef could only lead to the most terrifying conclusions.

'It's not the cows that are mad, it's the people' proclaimed an exasperated Dorrell, surveying the damage wrought on British agriculture—and the balance of trade—a week after his parliamentary statement. But the mad cow panic of March 1996 did not begin on the farms or in the butchers and supermarkets. It began among the scientists, spread to the politicians and was amplified in their interactions with the media, which transmitted it to the public. Nobody was better placed to dampen down the panic than Dorrell, yet he did more than anybody to promote the madness that devastated farmers in Britain and beyond. By September 1996 when the number of cases of nvCJD had reached fourteen, the mad cow panic had destroyed jobs and livelihoods numbered in thousands.

'We're in complete despair', said Fred Warner, nuclear scientist and visiting professor at Essex University's Scientific Committee on Problems of the Environment, 'if you look at the risks, you are more likely to be killed when you go out of your front door by a motor car than by Mad Cow Disease' (*The Times Higher Education Supplement*, 5 April). To grasp the impact of the mad cow panic, it is necessary to look more deeply into the psychopathology of the 'risk society'.

RISK SOCIETY

The panic about Mad Cow Disease took off in a society which has become preoccupied with collective fears of impending doom and with individual anxieties about threats to health, security and safety. We worry about nuclear war and global warming, AIDS and Ebola, mugging and burglary, road rage, child abuse and violence against women. The collapse of established frameworks in the fields of economics, politics and morality has created a uniquely insecure society (see Furedi 1997).

As we have seen, the effects of the collective anxiety neurosis can be discerned even amongst the most hard-headed scientists and politicians. Even the epidemiologists who argued in November 1995 that the evidence did not show a link between BSE and CJD felt obliged to add 'but, unfortunately, it does not strongly reject that possibility either' (Hofmans and Wientjens 1995). The absurd demand for conclusive proof that BSE does *not* cause CJD was endlessly repeated by politicians and journalists.

The peculiar difficulty of proving that something does *not* cause something else arises from the presumption that some familiar activity—like eating beef, walking down the street, driving to work, breathing—should now be assumed to be of lethal danger unless proved otherwise. This is indeed a crazy world, one in which all men are potential rapists and child abusers, all strangers dangerous and all encounters with the natural environment imminently life-threatening.

In normal times people accept that there are risks in everyday life, take routine steps to avoid them, and carry on with their lives. But we are not living in normal times. Today a morbid anxiety permeates society, inflating risks and demanding a level of reassurance that can never be achieved. The very indeterminacy of the risks that preoccupy people provides full scope for the upsurge of irrational fears.

An editorial in *The Guardian* in response to the December 1995 scare illustrates the mindset of the risk society ('Mad cows and Englishmen', 8 December). It acknowledged that 'there may not be a link' between BSE and CJD, but insisted that 'there are genuine worries':

> People who ate infected meat in the late 1980s may not show signs of the disease until way into the next millenium. Then, if the doomsday scenario proved right, biblical numbers could suffer loss of coordination, intellect and personality—just like the wobbly mad cows seen on television.

Though it was not explained what intellectual impairment or personality changes were experienced by those cows, the drift was clear.

Proceeding from the (then unsubstantiated) presumption that 'infected meat' could cause CJD, within a few sentences the editorial was speculating about dementia and death on a biblical scale. When confronted with the absurdity of such a scenario, panic promoters take refuge in indeterminacy —'it could happen', 'unlikely perhaps, but not impossible', 'you can never be certain'. This sequence, reinforced by scary images of wobbly mad cows, leads inexorably to the familiar cautions that 'you can't be too careful', 'better safe than sorry', and the advice that you should stop whatever everyday activity is linked to the latest risk that has been discovered.

If you cannot prove with mathematical certainty that beef is safe, then, the logic runs, the sensible course of action is to stop eating it. However, as consumer experts hastened to advise us, this is by no means as straightforward as it might seem. Potentially brain-curdling beef products find their way into cakes, puddings, biscuits, even gelatin drug capsules and fruit gums. Avoiding beef requires a high level of vigilance and close attention to the small print on food packaging.

An alternative course of action is to eat only beef produced by organic farmers. But, as another helpful *The Guardian* article explained, this too requires considerable effort:

> Go to a butcher who is knowledgeable and committed to selling organic meat. Find out which farm he gets his beef from and check that with a list of organic farms provided by the Soil Association (16 December).

Another alternative would be to get a bullock (from an approved organic farm of course) for your garden or allotment—perhaps the Soil Association provides a DIY slaughtering guide.

The price of the mad cow panic is not only the extra cost of these alternatives but the cost in time and energy spent in reading food packages, checking out butchers and working out alternatives to beef. Ironically, the resulting dementia may prove even more rapidly progressive than that of CJD.

The German sociologist Ulrich Beck, who pioneered the concept of the 'risk society', addressed a conference in Britain on 'The Politics of the Risk Society' at the height of the mad cow scare. Linking the issue of BSE and CJD to the nuclear leak at Chernobyl and the dangers of genetic engineering, Beck accused scientists of conducting experiments on society without knowing the consequences: 'neglecting risks', he suggested, was 'one of the most effective ways of reinforcing them' (*The Independent*, 1 April). Beck emphasizes uncertainty to create an enhanced sense of risk which he then deploys to cast doubt on the value of social and scientific progress. His thesis is premised on the ultimate worst-case scenario—human extinction:

> I use the term 'risk society' for those societies that are confronted by the challenges of the self-created possibility, hidden at first, then increasingly apparent, of the self-destruction of all life on this earth.

The abstract postulation of extinction gives Beck licence to discuss all innovations in a tone of impending doom and to inflate all known risks to humanity.

The logic of Beck's argument is that nothing new should be tried, since the risks involved cannot be foreseen. Anybody who recommends change must first prove that it will be safe. Indeed this approach—dignified as the 'precautionary principle' and enthusiastically promoted by environmentalists—has become an increasingly influential theme in modern society. But, since the full consequences of any change can never be known in advance, the implementation of this principle would prevent any form of scientific or social experimentation. As Furedi argues in *Culture of Fear: Risk-taking and the morality of low expectations*, 'by institutionalizing caution, the precautionary principle imposes a doctrine of limits':

> It offers security, but in exchange for lowering expectations, limiting growth and preventing experimentation and change (Furedi 1997).

In the 'risk society' caution is elevated to become the prime directive of human action.

The popular argument that British society has been subjected to an experiment to discover the transmissibility of BSE to human beings (a Horizon documentary on BSE/CJD broadcast by the BBC in November 1996 was entitled 'The human experiment') contains elements of falsehood and truth. It is false in the sense that the term 'experiment' implies a conscious strategy of exposing humans to BSE so that the results could be studied, an allegation which has not emerged from even the most paranoid of the BSE dissidents. It is true in the sense that nvCJD appears to be the unexpected consequence of innovations in cattle feeding in the 1970s and 1980s, which first gave rise to BSE.

What conclusions should be drawn from this experience of an experiment that went wrong? For those for whom the whole concept of experiment has become anathema, the conclusion is that we should regress from modern to more primitive agricultural techniques, though they are rarely explicit about how far back they think we should go. For those of us who cling to the spirit of experimentation, the conclusion is that we should do what humanity has done in the past—learn the lessons of this unfortunate experience, deal with its unexpected consequences and move on.

The history of medicine reveals countless examples of experiments with disastrous results yielding insights for future innovations. Take the history of blood transfusion or major organ transplantation. Early experiments provoked public alarums—and carried a 100% fatality rate. Thanks in part to these and further experiments, yielding a deeper understanding of tissue compatability, both techniques are in routine use, enhancing the quantity and quality of human lives. One of the most damaging aspects of the precautionary principle is that it robs us of any chance of learning from our mistakes and thus condemns us to a relentless cycle of regression.

THE REVENGE OF NATURE

'Is it altogether fanciful to see the threat of a major outbreak of CJD as a symptom of nature's rebellion against human hubris?' asked Oxford philosopher John Gray in a polemical response to the March ministerial statements entitled 'Nature bites back' (*The Guardian*, 26 March). The theme that the new cases of CJD represented the revenge of nature against human interference in the form of intensive farming methods, such as the feeding of meat products to herbivores, in defiance of 'natural laws', had considerable popular appeal.

Yet there is no basis to the claim that 'unnatural' practices carry greater risks (Gillott 1996). On the contrary: the development of science and technology through systematic interference in nature has not only equipped us to overcome many of the problems which dogged humanity in the past, but has also given us the capacity to cope with new problems as they arise.

Take the example of modern farming methods. Environmentalist sentimentality nothwithstanding, there is no such thing as a 'natural' method of farming. Agriculture is by definition a violation of nature. Its development ten thousand years ago marked one of the first great triumphs of humanity over nature and a key step towards a civilized society. Every advance in farming since has been achieved by overcoming natural barriers.

The American environmentalist Jeremy Rifkin claims that problems like BSE have arisen because we have 'denatured' cattle (Rifkin 1996).

But cattle are the creations of human ingenuity—the result of centuries of deliberate breeding according to human requirements, of 'denaturing' nature. There is little natural about any aspect of cattle farming. To get dairy cows to produce milk, calves are taken away from them immediately after birth. All cattle, whether they are destined to produce milk or meat, need more food than they would get on open pasture if they are to produce the quality and quantity of foodstuffs we require. Whether farmers use clover and hay, soya and silage, or animal-based feeds, all are 'unnatural' methods dictated by human needs.

The controversy about 'turning cows into cannibals'—because they were fed with the products of cattle offal as well as that from sheep and other species—has raged around the mad cow panic. But this is irrational. Cattle may customarily eat grass, but like most mammals they are omnivores, quite capable of digesting animal as well as plant protein. Indeed feeding animal protein to cattle long predates modern intensive farming. In the past it has taken many different forms, including the feeding of fish meal and fertilizer made of crushed bones, offal and blood.

Animal husbandry, like many aspects of human advance, has always created problems as well as bringing benefits. Many familiar infectious diseases became established in human society through close contact with domestic animals. Yet the wider progress achieved in part through the advance of agriculture has enabled human society (largely) to transcend the limitations imposed by infectious epidemics. The striking feature of modern society is that we face much less of a threat from nature than at any time in human history. While modern innovations may still give rise to unforeseen problems, our capacity to deal with these problems is much greater than in the past. The rapid detection and containment of BSE is a good example.

The popularity of the notion that the source of all our problems lies in the very attempt to increase human control over nature reveals the deep despondency of modern society and its extraordinary collapse of confidence in itself.

TRUST NOBODY

One of the key factors underlying the mad cow panic is the widespread conviction that government ministers cannot be trusted to tell the truth about the health risks associated with beef. A distrust for scientific and medical experts follows close behind the cynicism about politicians. Opinion polls confirm high levels of support for the view that the government and its expert advisers concealed information about the dangers of BSE to humans. According to an ICM poll for *The Guardian*, published on 3 April, 73% of people believed that 'the government knew there was a risk and tried to hide it', while 17% thought that it took prompt action as soon as it discovered the risk. Many believed that the government, because of party political and financial concerns, colluded with the beef trade and the farmers against the interests of consumers. Consumer groups, notably the Consumer Association, called for an 'independent inquiry' and for more information, notably in the form of labels on food products revealing their beef content, so that consumers could make 'informed choices' about what to eat (see *Health Which*, June 1996).

Popular scepticism about politicians and scientists contains many ironies. People who express utter cynicism about government ministers and SEAC are ready to put their faith in opposition politicians and critics like Lacey (who was formerly a British government and WHO adviser) and Dealler (who has now been brought into SEAC). Another striking feature of the distrust of official statements is that people almost invariably believe that the danger is even greater than has been admitted; they never seem to accuse the government of exaggerating risks. The rule of thumb appears to be that the more you distrust the government, the more you believe the panic: thus headlines in the far left *Socialist Worker* accused 'Crazy Tories' of 'wrecking our lives' and demanded 'Ban Beef Now!'. Yet from AIDS to BSE, the official record is one of consistently hyping up risks.

Furthermore, while echoing popular cyncism about politicians, the usual alternative recommended by radical critics of the government's record on BSE is to put our trust in some quango of government-appointed experts or in an even more anonymous and unaccountable agency responsible for labelling food products. Instead of questioning the scare, this approach amplifies anxieties—implying that the risks may be even greater than the government admits—and offers illusory solutions.

The very fact that radical scepticism about the statements of government ministers can be so readily allayed through the establishment of an inquiry or the provision of more information, reveals its superficiality. In fact, such scepticism is more a manifestation of a wider culture of mistrust than a specific questioning of governmental authority. The result is to reinforce the notion that that everyday life is full of mortal hazards, and that you cannot trust anybody, not the government, not the scientists, in the end, not even yourself. The outcome of this process is universal paranoia and paralysis.

CONCLUSION

Though there now appears to be a connection between BSE and nvCJD, many questions remain to be answered. There is still uncertainty over the origin of BSE and its mode of transmission and the likely course of the epidemic in cattle remains unclear. There are questions about the quantity of infective tissue required to transmit the infection, about the infectivity of other tissues apart from brain and spinal cord, about the possiblity of infectivity accumulating. Most importantly, the question of how many more will succumb to nvCJD is impossible to answer, though the small number of additional cases that have been confirmed in 1996 and early 1997 (bringing the total up to nineteen by June) must give grounds for optimism. Detailed investigation of the cases so far has failed to reveal whether particular individuals are more susceptible to this disease and why.

Indeed, though there has been a rapid advance in the understanding of the pathogenesis of prion diseases, notably at the level of molecular genetics, the function of the prion protein itself remains obscure. Fortunately, scientists like Collinge and his team stayed in their labs, and carried on with the serious research that is required to discover the exact nature of the link between BSE and CJD and the real risks of transmission. As Collinge emphasizes, this work already promises a test for early diagnosis of nvCJD as well as the beginnings of an approach towards therapeutic intervention. Thus science staggers on, even in a society in which it is more likely to provoke hostility than enthusiasm.

Given the present state of knowledge, there is nothing more we can now do to prevent the development of nvCJD in people who may have been exposed in the 1980s and are currently incubating the disease (Ridley and Baker, October 1996). We can, however, perceive the damage wrought by the mad cow panic and identify the forces that allowed it to gather momentum. The elevation of risk, the denigration of human intervention in nature and the culture of distrust all point towards making caution and restraint the guiding principles of society. Yet the surest way for us to feel swamped by the problems of modern society is to stop trying to do anything about them.

REFERENCES

Almond, J.W. et al. (November 1996) 'CJD and BSE: Any connection?' British Medical Journal, 311, 1415-21 (25 November).

Baker, H.F. and Ridley, R.M. (1988), 'BSE'. British Medical Journal, (9 July).

Blanchfield, J.R. (1996) 'Institute of Food Science and Technology position statement on BSE: Update of 29 October 1996'; 'promed' file 'bse-ifst'-961029. IFST website: http//www.easynet.co.uk/ifst/

Brown, P. (November 1995) 'The jury is still out'. British Medical Journal, 311, 1416 (25 November).

Brown, P. (March 1996) 'BSE and CJD'. British Medical Journal, 312, 790-1 (30 March).

Collee, J.G. (1991) Reply to Dealler and Lacey (Letter). The Lancet, 337, 173-4 (19 January).

Collinge, J. et al. (December 1995) 'Unaltered susceptibility to BSE in transgenic mice expressing human prion protein'. Nature, 318, 779 (21-28 December).

Collinge, J. et al. (October 1996) 'Molecular analysis of prion strain variation and the aetiology of "new variant" CJD'. Nature, 383, 685-690 (24 October).

Dealler, S. and Lacey, R. (1991) 'Beef and BSE: the risk persists'. Nutrition and Health, 7, 117-133.

Dealler, S. and Lacey, R. (1991) BSE and man (letter). The Lancet, 337, 173 (19 January).

Dealler, S. (1996) Lethal Legacy: BSE—the search for the truth. London, Bloomsbury.

Fitzpatrick, M. (February 1996) 'A mad, mad, mad, mad world'. Living Marxism, 87, pp14-17.

Fitzpatrick, M. (April 1996) 'More mad cow madness—a GP's view'. Public Health News, 7, 4, 53-54.

Fitzpatrick, M. (April 1996) 'CJD and BSE: Scientists who inflame public anxieties must share responsibility of resulting panic'. British Medical Journal, 312, 1037 (20 April).

Fitzpatrick, M. (May 1996) 'The great mad cow panic'. Living Marxism, 90, pp24-27.

Ford, B. (1996) BSE: The facts—Mad Cow Disease and the risk to mankind. London, Corgi.

Furedi, F. (1997) Culture of Fear: Risk-taking and the morality of low expectations. London, Cassell.

Gillott, J. (1996) 'Who's afraid of nature's revenge?'. Living Marxism, 90, pp 28-30.

Gore, S. (November 1995) 'More than happenstance: CJD in farmers and young adults'. British Medical Journal, 311, 1416 (25 November).

Gore, S .(March 1996) 'Bovine CJD?', British Medical Journal. 312, 791-2 (30 March).

Hofman, A. and Wientjens, D. (1995) 'Epidemiological evidence concerning a possible causal link'. British Medical Journal, 311, 1418-19 (25 November).

Hoinville, L.J. et al. (1995) 'An investigation of risk factors for cases of BSE born after the introduction of the feed ban'. Veterinary Record, 136, 312-318.

Holt, T.A. and Phillips, J (1988) 'BSE'. British Medical Journal, 531 (4 June).

Lacey, R. (1994) <u>Mad Cow Disease: The history of BSE in Britain</u>. Saint Helier, Jersey, Gypsela.

Lacey, R. (1996) 'MAFF hears what it wants to hear'. <u>The Times Higher Education Supplement</u>, 29 March.

Lawson, Mark (1996) 'Icebergs and rocks and the "good" lie', <u>The Guardian</u>, 24 June.

Ridley, R.M. (1995) Review of Lacey, R (1994) 'Mad Cow Disease: The history of BSE in Britain'. <u>British Medical Journal</u>, **311**, 67-8, 1 July.

Ridley, R.M. and Baker, H.F. (1995) 'The myth of maternal transmission of spongiform encephalopathy'. <u>British Medical Journal</u>, **311**, 1071-76 (21 October).

Ridley, R.M. and Baker, H.F. (October 1996) Oral transmission of BSE to primates. <u>The Lancet</u>, **348,** 9035 (26 October).

Rifkin, J. (1996) <u>Beyond Beef: The rise and fall of the cattle culture</u>. Thorsons.

Southwood, R (1989) <u>Report of the Working Party on BSE</u>. London, HMSO.

Will, R. et al. (April 1996) 'A new variant of CJD in the United Kingdom'. <u>The Lancet</u>, **347**, 921-25 (6 April).

Part Two

Science and Social Science:
Evaluating Risks

CREUTZFELDT-JAKOB DISEASE: RARE TRANSMISSIBLE SPONGIFORM ENCEPHALOPATHY WITH AN IMPORTANT MESSAGE

Colin L. Masters

It would have been difficult to predict the magnitude of the problem created when attention was drawn to a possible causal association between BSE and the emergence of nvCJD (Will et al. 1996). With hindsight, of course, it is possible to make suggestions on how this could have been better managed so that the economic impact would have been minimized. But the underlying medical, scientific and public health issues remain dauntingly complex. I set out below some of the principles which form the basis of our current understanding of this group of diseases (Table 1).

TABLE 1: **TRANSMISSIBLE SPONGIFORM ENCEPHALOPATHIES**

Disease	Natural Host
scrapie	sheep and goats
transmissible mink encephalopathy (TME)	mink
chronic wasting disease (CWD)	mule deer and elk
bovine spongiform encephalopathy (BSE)	cattle
feline spongiform encephalopathy (FSE)	cats, cheetah
exotic ungulate encephalopathy (EUE)	nyala
kuru	humans - Fore
Creutzfeldt-Jakob disease (CJD)	humans
Gerstmann-Sträussler-Scheinker syndrome (GSS)	humans
fatal familial insomnia (FFI)	humans

As a keen observer (our laboratory maintains a comprehensive if not definitive bibliography on CJD and related conditions) and sometime participant in this field over the last thirty years, the major lesson I have learned is that the study of rare and esoteric disease entities may often provide some fundamental insights of wide applicability. For some recent reviews of this area, see Aguzzi et al. (1997), Bamborough et al. (1996), Caughey and Chesebro (1997), DeArmond and Prusiner (1997), Hoarwich and Weissmann (1997), Ironside et al. (1996), Prusiner (1996), Weissmann (1996), Wickner et al. (1996).

A BRIEF HISTORY

Scrapie, endemic in sheep and goats in Europe and North America, had long been known to be an infectious disease, beginning with observations in the eighteenth century. H. Creutzfeldt and A. Jakob described the occurrence of subacute neurodegenerative illnesses in a series of patients, the first report appearing in 1920. We have had an opportunity to review the slides of Jakob's cases (Masters and Gajdusek 1982) and conclude that indeed some of Jakob's cases would still be accepted as *bona fide* examples of subacute spongiform encephalopathies, as judged by contemporary criteria. While some doubt will always remain over the nature of Creutzfeldt's case, the eponym of Creutzfeldt-Jakob disease has become established and entrenched. Kuru, first described in the western scientific literature by Gajdusek and Zigas (1957), occurred in a restricted population of Eastern Highlanders in Papua New Guinea. The disease had reached hyper-endemic proportions by the time of European contact, when it was the major cause of death of women and children.

After the pathologic description of kuru was published, a link was drawn to sheep scrapie (Hadlow 1959). Confirmation came when the transmissbility of kuru to non-human primates was demonstrated: direct intracerebral inoculation of kuru brain to a chimpanzee caused disease after a long incubation period (Gajdusek et al. 1966). This was quickly followed by the evidence that CJD was also transmissible (Gibbs et al. 1968), opening a new era of research into the nature of the infectious agents responsible for these diseases.

EPIDEMIOLOGY

There are three principal forms of CJD: sporadic, inherited and acquired. The sporadic form occurs world-wide at an annual rate of one per million population, and accounts for the majority (greater than 90%) of all cases. The mean age at death is fifty-five to sixty years, and most cases succumb to an illness which lasts less than ten months. Clinically, the neurologic manifestations are widespread with involvement of all major systems (diffuse neocortical, corticospinal, extrapyramidal and cerebellar systems) with the principal feature of subacute progressive dementia accompanied by myoclonus. Less commonly, one of the neurologic systems appears to take the brunt of the illness (e.g. the Heidenhein variant with occipital cortical involvement). Pathologically, the typical triad of spongiform change, gliosis and neuronal loss is seen by conventional light microscopy.

The inherited forms of CJD occur in an autosomal dominantly transmitted pattern with almost complete penetrance. Their ages at onset are slightly younger than sporadic cases. In every pedigree studied to date, a pathogenic mutation has been identified in the

PRNP gene (the gene which codes the for the prion protein, PrP). As far as can be determined, these inherited forms of CJD are as infectious as the sporadic forms—thus creating a totally novel class of inherited infectious disease. Geographic clusters of familial disease have been observed.

The acquired forms of CJD are of increasing importance. Iatrogenic transmission of CJD is now well recognized, through contaminated tissue transplants (cornea, dura mater), neurosurgical instruments (including stereotaxic depth electrodes) and extracts of hormones derived from human pituitaries (growth hormone and gonadotrophin). These iatrogenic forms of CJD now total nearly two hundred cases. The prolonged incubation periods (often more than a decade) after peripheral or low-dose contamination are consistent with a large body of experimental evidence. A review of the PRNP genotype of iatrogenic cases shows that homozygosity at codon one hundred and twenty-nine may be a predisposing risk factor.

This raises important questions for those cases of sporadic CJD in whom a similar homozygosity is demonstrated—do they represent an unrecognized contamination event? Despite considerable epidemiological studies, most cases of sporadic CJD do not demonstrate any other risk factor, while some studies have shown an excess of surgical procedures in the ten years prior to onset. Occupational history (especially in the health industry), education, diet, travel histories, exposure to blood transfusions have been studied, without positive associations being determined.

The progressive disappearance of kuru since 1960 has been most instructive. The dramatic rate of disappearance appears to have followed an exponentially decreasing curve. Today, nearly forty years after the cessation of the contamination events (cannibalism), cases are still occurring with a frequency which far exceeds the sporadic background level (i.e. one in a million). Within a decade, we will know whether the incubation period can match or even exceed the normal human life expectancy.

Were it not for the outbreak of BSE in the United Kingdom in 1985/1986, scrapie would have remained the subject of investigation of only a handful of dedicated scientists. The rapidity with which BSE spread within the English dairy herd surprised everyone, and indicated that a major contamination event had occurred approximately eight years earlier. Fortunately, the veterinary epidemiologists suspected transmission through contaminated stock food derived from rendered ruminant meat and bone meal. The introduction of progressive bans of feeding ruminant materials to ruminants and other livestock has slowly brought the epidemic under control. The striking similarities between this outbreak and the phenomenon of kuru are obvious. The rate at which BSE can be completely eliminated from the bovine population will now depend on factors such as low level contamination within the actual environment of the population at risk, and on the remote possibility of vertical (transplacental) transmission. While the kuru experience would speak strongly against the possibility of maternal transmission, the problem of low level environmental contamination with incubation periods which may exceed the normal life expectancy of a cow is a formidable challenge.

MOLECULAR PATHOGENESIS OF INFECTIVITY

Three independent and converging lines of study provide the compelling evidence that PrP lies at the center of this disease. First, PrP co-purifies with infectivity (Bolton et al. 1982). Second, the amyloid plaques characteristic of some forms of CJD and scrapie are composed of PrP filamentous aggregates (Prusiner et al. 1983). Third, a variety of mutations in PRNP cause CJD (Hsiao et al. 1989). Each of these three lines of evidence has been extensively elaborated by Prusiner, and for this he was awarded the 1997 Nobel Prize in Physiology or Medicine.

The conversion of normal host PrP^C (the normal isoform of PrP) to the disease-associated form ($PrP^{SC/CJD}$) is operationally defined on the basis of relative protease resistance and a change in conformation from α-helix to β-sheet. The accumulation of PrP^{SC} (the scrapie isoform of PrP) in the diseased brain is thought to underlie the infectious nature of this disease, although the minimal infectious unit has not yet been defined. Additional modifying molecules (a postulated 'protein-X') also remain undefined. The slow kinetics of replication and the absence of any host immune response are readily explained by the conversion of PrP^C by either a template-directed or nucleated/seeding crystallization (see Figure 1). The mechanism of neuronal degeneration (and vacuolation) caused by $PrP^{SC/CJD}$ remains uncertain, as does the normal function of the PrP molecule itself.

Rational therapeutic approaches are now being explored, based on this understanding of molecular pathogenesis. If the conversion of PrP^C to PrP^{SC} can be altered, or if the toxic property of the PrP^{SC} aggregate can be inhibited, then a therapy for this class of infectious disease can be envisioned. Indeed, preliminary *in vitro* assays have already suggested that lead compounds with the amyloid-binding qualities found for Congo Red, doxirubicin, or sulfated polyanions might be useful.

THE EMERGENCE OF nvCJD—THE FIRST ZOONOTIC TRANSMISSION OF CJD

In March 1996, the United Kingdom CJD Surveillance Unit advised their government that there could be a link between BSE and a newly recognized variant form of CJD. In the preceding two years, a series of eleven cases of CJD had been seen with unusual clinical and pathologic features. Clinically, the cases were young (some in teenagers), presenting with psychiatric symptoms, sensory disturbances, early cerebellar signs, late dementia, long duration (greater than twelve months) and lack of typical EEG changes. Pathologically, the defining features were an unusual and abundant deposition of PrP amyloid ('florid' plaques) with prominent involvement of the basal ganglia. While clinically some features were reminiscent of kuru, pathologically the features were quite distinct.

Over the past two years, the total number of confirmed cases has risen to twenty-eight. There is now compelling molecular and experimental evidence that this new variant CJD is indeed closely related to BSE (Bruce et al. 1997). All cases have been homozygous at codon one hundred and twenty-nine of PRNP. It is possible that these cases represent the highest genetic susceptibility group within the population, and that the heterozygotes will follow in the future. These present cases are presumed to have acquired their infections at least ten years previously. The maximal contamination of the human food chain with BSE probably occurred between 1982 and 1987. Intense epidemiologic studies of these nvCJD cases have failed to identify any environmental risk factor which could account for their occurrence.

While the bovine disease appears to be coming under control, a very large question mark hangs over the future extent of the spread of this disease into the human population. At one extreme, the low infectiousness of CJD caused by the species barrier and a very peripheral route of inoculation could combine to limit the number of human cases to only a few more than presently ascertained. At the other extreme, a large proportion of the European population has been exposed to a wide variety of products contaminated with the BSE agent. At this time it is impossible to predict what the final outcome will look like.

FIGURE 1

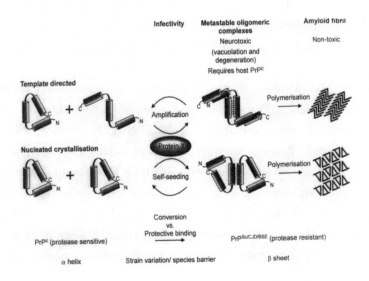

FIGURE LEGEND

Two hypotheses attempt to explain the phenomenon of a self-replicating infectious protein. In the template directed model, the normal isoform of PrP (shown here as a triangular shaped back-bone resembling the α-helical domains) encounters an abnormal conformer of PrP. This process engenders a metastable oligomeric complex in which the normal isomer is induced to assume a similar conformation. The forward conversion reaction is either modulated by 'protein-X' or the abnormal conformer is maintained by 'protein-X'. Disease results from the toxic effect of the metastable complex. Further polymerization of the complex may result in amyloid fibril formation.

For the nucleated crystallization model, the self-seeded oligomeric complex is more dependent on the self-perpetuating properties of the oligomeric complex, which may also result in amyloid fibril formation. Both hypotheses require the operational conversion of PrP^C (protease sensitive, predominantly α-helical) to PrP^{SC} (protease resistant, predominantly β-sheet). In both hypotheses, there is an absolute requirement for PrP^C to maintain the cycle of conversion, and hence, infectivity.

REFERENCES

Aguzzi, A., Bitiftler, T., Klein, M., Brandner, S., Raeber, A., Flechsig, E., Weissmann, C., Neurotoxicity and neuroinvasiveness of prions. Brain Pathology, 1997; 7, 1137-1138.

Bamborough, P., Wille, H., Telling, G.C., Yehiely, F., Prusiner, S.B., Cohen, F.E., Prion protein structure and scrapie replication—theoretical, spectroscopic, and genetic investigations. Cold Spring Harbor Symposia on Quantitative Biology, 1996; 61:495-509.

Bolton, D.C., McKinley, M.P., Prusiner, S.B., Identification of a protein that purifies with the scrapie prion. Science, 1982; 218:1309-1311.

Bruce, M.E., Will, R.G., Ironside, J.W. et al., Transmissions to mice indicate that 'new variant' CJD is caused by the BSE agent. Nature, 1997; 389:498-501.

Caughey, B., Chesebro, B., Prion protein and the transmissible spongiform encephalopathies. Trends in Cell Biology, 1997; 7:56-62.

DeArmond, S.J., Prusiner, S.B., Prion diseases. In: Graham, D.I., Lantos, P.L., eds,

Greenfield's Neuropathology, 6th ed. London:Arnold,1997: 235-280.

Gajdusek, D.C., Gibbs, C.J. Jr., Alpers, M., Experimental transmission of a kuru-like syndrome to chimpanzees. Nature, 1966; 209:794-796.

Gajdusek, D.C., Zigas, V., Degenerative disease of the central nervous system in New Guinea. The endemic occurrence of 'kuru' in the native population. New England Journal of Medicine, 1957; 257:974-978.

Gibbs, C.J. Jr., Gajdusek, D.C., Asher, D.M., Alpers, M.P., Beck, E., Daniel, P.M., Matthews, W.B., Creutzfeldt-Jakob disease (spongiform encephalopathy): transmission to the chimpanzee. Science, 1968; 161: 388-389.

Hadlow, W.J., Scrapie and kuru. The Lancet, 1959; 2:289-290.

Hsiao, K., Baker, H.F., Crow, T.J., Poulter, M., Owen, F., Terwilliger, J.D., Westaway, D., Ott, J., Prusiner, S.B., Linkage of a prion protein missense variant to Gerstmann-Sträussler syndrome. Nature, 1989; 338:342-345.

Horwich, A.L., Weissman, J.S., Deadly conformations: Protein misfolding in prion disease. Cell, 1997; 89:499-510.

Ironside, J.W., Sutherland, K., Bell, J.E., McCardle, L., Barrie, C., Estebeiro, K., Zeidler, M., Will, R.G., A new variant of Creutzfeldt-Jakob disease—neuropathological and clinical features. Cold Spring Harbor Symposia on Quantitative Biology, 1996; 61:523-530.

Masters, C.L., Gajdusek, D.C., The spectrum of Creutzfeldt-Jakob disease and the virus-induced subacute spongiform encephalopathies. In: Smith WT and Cavanagh JB, editors. Recent Advances in Neuropathology. Churchill Livingstone, Edinburgh, Chapter 6, 1982; 2:139-163.

Prusiner, S.B., Molecular biology and genetics of prion diseases. Cold Spring Harbor Symposia on Quantitative Biology, 1996; 61:473-493.

Prusiner, S.B., McKinley, M.P., Bowman, K.A., Bolton, D.C., Bendheim, P.E., Groth, D.F., Glenner, G.G., Scrapie prions aggregate to form amyloid-like birefringent rods. Cell, 1983; 35:349-358.

Weissmann, C., Molecular biology of transmissible spongiform encephalopathies. FEBS Lett, 1996; 389:3-11.

Wickner, R.B., Masison, D.C., Edskes, H.K., Maddelein, M.L. Prions of yeast, [PSI] and [URE3], as models for neurodegenerative diseases. Cold Spring Harbor Symposia on Quantitative Biology, 1996; 61:541-550.

Will, R.G., Ironside, J.W., Zeidler, M., Cousens, S.N., Estibeiro, K., Alperovitch, A., Poser, S., Pocchiari, M., Hofman, A., Smith, P.G. A new variant of Creutzfeldt-Jakob disease in the UK. The Lancet, 1996; 347:921-925.

RISK ASSESSMENT AND CREUTZFELDT-JAKOB DISEASE
Simon Grant

INTRODUCTION

Q1 Who drove a car to attend work this morning?

Q2 Of those who answered yes, who would refuse a plate of English (beef) steak?

Both of these questions involve decisions made under uncertainty. Given the best available scientific evidence (reinforced by Professor Master's article in this book) the former involves much higher probabilities of serious injury and possible death than the latter. Yet many of you (and I would include myself) are quite willing to accept the risks associated with driving a car, but not those with eating English beef.

Q3 How should we think about these decisions? Are we making rational assessments about the risks involved? Is the current furore over British beef an over-reaction, a panic?

As Simon Jenkin wrote in *The Times*, reprinted in *The Australian*, April 28 1996:

> Last December the scientists told them that beef was safe. There was no evidence of a link between a dwindling outbreak of BSE and a few random cases of human CJD. They put the adjective 'inconceivable'

before the much abused word risk. Ministers took their word for it and cheered.

Now on the basis of the same clinical evidence (or lack of it), the scientists say that they are not so sure. They have put the word inconceivable in a test tube, added a coincidence or two, heated them to hysteria point and produced a rather different adjective: extremely small.

What have been the consequences? A collapse in consumer confidence in Britain and abroad in beef and a world-wide export ban on United Kingdom beef imposed by the European Union. The financial costs of the agreed partial cull have been estimated to be approximately seven hundred million dollars per year (over the next five to six years) plus a 20% fall in British beef output, reducing Gross Domestic Product (GDP) by a small percentage (0.05%), with hopefully few jobs lost. But there still exists the spectre of a full cull that would cost in total around twenty billion dollars; pose a threat to four hundred thousand jobs in the beef and associated industries; and precipitate a fall in GDP of around 1.2%.

Is this an over-reaction? It is interesting to note that Europe's panic about this vague prospect of a CJD epidemic overshadowed a warning from WHO that the world faced a threat from tuberculosis, a disease the developed world believed it had conquered. WHO said tuberculosis could kill thirty million people in the next decade.

I am an economist. To be more specific a micro-economic theorist, specializing in decision making under uncertainty. It is usual for economists when analyzing social interactions such as the market for beef to model the decision makers therein as *rational* actors. What do I mean by that? Essentially I mean that the decision maker has well-defined goals or aims (that is, preferences) and understands the environmental and economic constraints that she or he faces. Out of the available alternatives, the decision maker chooses the best according to her goals or aims (according to her preferences). From these individual decisions we build up a theory of aggregate behaviour for our society. It is not that we literally believe that people are the super-rational maximizing automata of our theory but rather that such an abstraction of people's identity and motivations is useful in our branch of social analysis.

What I wish to argue, is that it is undoubtedly true that our individual cognitive abilities are flawed and may exhibit systematic biases. However, the current crisis in consumer confidence in British beef that stemmed from the British government's announcement in March 1996 admitting a possible link between BSE in cows and a variant of CJD in humans can be explained within a model of perfectly rational agents. Moreover, that it is useful to do so, as it provides insights as to how best to proceed and avoid such crises in the future.

RATIONAL CHOICE THEORY

When I studied Economics 1, at the Australian National University back in 1982, the lecturer introduced the theory of rational choice with an example of a consumer dividing her expenditure between two goods, beer and pies. What the consumer chose, that is, the optimal combination of pies and beer given the amount of money she had available to expend, was concrete in the sense that this was the bundle of goods that she would physically consume.

Now the theory is very flexible and can readily be extended to incorporate: many goods; temporal choice, that is consumption today versus consumption tomorrow; and even choice under uncertainty, where the trade-off is between consumption given that one state of the world obtains versus consumption given that another state of the world obtains.

In the last case what I am choosing among are 'contingent' bundles. At the time of my choice I do not know what I will end up experiencing. For example, in deciding whether to take out fire insurance, if I don't take out the insurance then how much I consume depends upon whether the items that were to be insured are destroyed by fire or not. Returning to my original two questions, by deciding to drive my car here this morning what I end up experiencing depends upon whether I have an accident or not. If I consume the plate of English beef, I may view it as conceivable that I could contract CJD and die an untimely and unpleasant death.

When dealing with decision making under uncertainty economists and many other social scientists typically employ the theory of Subjective Expected Utility that was rigorously formulated by a statistician, Leonard Savage, at the University of Chicago. A pre-eminent economic theorist at Stanford University, David Kreps, has described Savage's Subjective Expected Utility theory as the 'crowning jewel of choice theory'. Part of this theory entails that decision makers have well structured beliefs about the likelihood of any contingency that may arise from any decision that is available to them. Formally these beliefs can be quantified as mathematical probabilities. In the next section I shall briefly mention some results from the psychology literature that addresses the question of how well actual individual's judgements about likelihoods of uncertain events conform to a mathematical probability distribution.

THE PSYCHOLOGY OF JUDGMENT UNDER UNCERTAINTY

When, as experts or lay persons, we think about and make judgments in the presence of uncertainty, we make use of heuristic procedures. In the ordinary run of events, these serve us very well, but at best they are only approximate and may sometimes lead to biased estimates or even outright errors. Psychologists have identified the following main heuristic procedures.

Availability—a probability judgment is driven by the ease with which they can think of previous occurrences of the event, or the ease with which they can imagine the event occurring. But a variety of factors can introduce bias when this heuristic is used. For example, in an experiment psychologists (Liechtenstein et al. 1978) told several groups of well educated Americans that roughly fifty thousand people die each year in traffic accidents. They were then asked to estimate the number of deaths that occur each year in the United States from a variety of other causes.

Deaths from botulism are quite rare but Americans learn through the press about virtually every one that occurs. Deaths from strokes are fairly common, but Americans typically learn about them only when a friend, relative or famous person is involved. If one plots the (average) estimated number of deaths vertically against the actuarially determined incidence rates, it is apparent that the incidence rate of causes such as botulism is overestimated and that of risks such as stroke is underestimated.

Anchoring and Adjustment—an anchor is selected as a first approximation, then this value is adjusted to reflect supplementary information. Typically, the adjustment is insufficient and the result is biased towards the anchor. The previous experiment was repeated except that subjects were told instead that about one thousand people die each year in the United States from accidental electrocutions. The operation of the heuristic of anchoring and adjustment is clearly illustrated by a systematic downward shift in all the resulting estimates.

Characterizing Risk Perceptions
Q What do people mean when they say something is risky?

Slovic, Fischhoff and Liechtenstein,[1] conducted a study to try to understand people's perceptions and predict societal response in a way useful for informing policy decisions. They asked individuals in four groups (experts, students, League of Women Voters, and Active Club members) to consider the *risk of dying* across United States society as a whole for thirty hazards. Risks rated least were given a rating of ten. After rating the risks each group judged the acceptability of the risk by specifying a risk-adjustment factor—whether (given perceived costs and benefits) a risk should be raised or lowered. They were then asked to rate the risk characteristics of each hazard on a seven point scale.

The characteristics were:
1. voluntariness of risk
2. immediacy of effect
3. knowledge about risk
4. known to science

5. control over risk
6. newness
7. chronic-catastrophic
8. common-dread
9. severity of consequence

These were found to be able to be grouped into two factors
1. Unknown Risk (Characteristics 1– 6)
2. Dread Risk (Characteristics 7–9)

Slovic, Fischhoff and Liechtenstein found that:
- judgments of risk characteristics were quite similar for all groups;
- for lay groups, perceived risk and desired magnitude of adjustment highly correlated with Dread Risk;
- experts' risk judgments did not correlate highly with any of the characteristics but rather were closely related to actuarially determined estimates of average annual fatalities for each activity; and
- judgments of desired regulatory stringency (made only by students) were related to Dread Risk.

It seems clear to me that experts and lay persons were answering different questions when quantifying their risk perceptions. Experts attempted to give their 'best' guess of actuarially determined incidence rates. The estimates of lay people seem confounded with their relative valuation of the consequence of a fatality resulting from that hazard or from simply *facing* the risk of that hazard. Similarly researchers in England have consistently found public willingness-to-pay for given reduction in the likelihood of fatality on public transport is many times greater than for the equivalent reduction in private transport and the authors of the study argue forcefully that it is quite rational for people to feel and act that way.

My guess is that the risk of contracting CJD from eating beef is high in both factors and that the public is keen for its reduction.

RATIONAL HERDS

So one might suggest that psychological biases account for the seemingly panicked response of the English beef-eating public to the statement in March admitting a possible link between BSE in cows and CJD in humans. The statement 'anchored' in the minds of the public focussing their attention on the possibility of this disease and inciting fear and dread.

However, I wish to propose a more 'rational actor' based explanation that relies on the recent development of the theory of 'rational herds' or 'informational cascade'.[2]

The starting point for these analyses is the observation that a striking regularity of human society is *localized conformity*. Four primary mechanisms have been suggested for uniform social behaviour:
1. sanctions on deviants;
2. positive payoff externalities—(e.g. common technical standard);
3. conformity preference—(driving on left-hand side or right-hand side of road is self-enforcing); and
4. communication—if costless and credible will lead to conformity on correct action.

None of these explanations, however, can explain why mass behaviour is often fragile in the sense that small shocks can frequently lead to large shifts in behaviour. Banerjee and Bikhchandani's theory offers an explanation not only of why people conform but also of why convergence of behaviour can be idiosyncratic and fragile. In their model, individuals rapidly converge on one action (say, avoid English beef) on the basis of some but very little information. The basic idea is that a 'herd' or 'informational cascade' occurs when it is optimal for an individual, having observed the actions of those ahead, to follow that behaviour regardless of his or her own information.

It seems clear that the British government took actions to reinforce the first cascade that 'beef is safe' (recall in 1990 the then United Kingdom Agriculture Minister, John Gummer, dismissing fears of human BSE infection from cattle by attempting to feed hamburger to his four-year-old daughter Cordelia in front of reporters). In 1995 there was a fresh scare as group of eminent scientists admitted they had stopped eating British beef. In 1996 after the government's admission, people stopped eating beef and others followed, including fast-food chains such as McDonald's who announced on 27 March that it had banned British beef from its burgers in Britain. In a statement, McDonald's said it had complete confidence in the safety of British beef but was taking the step to maintain consumer trust. Presumably its confidence was based on its own inspection regime but that information was lost in the 'whirl' of the informational cascade. An added complication with McDonald's is that it is not trying to maximize its own expectation of using beef but rather its expectation of the market's (rational) expectation of McDonald's using British beef. It is a subtle point but maximizing your expectation of the consequences of your action is not the same thing as maximizing your expectation of someone else's expectation of the consequences of your action. So inhibited, McDonald's was a rational response to a rational expectation of the market.

Reputation (public confidence) is a fragile asset. In such circumstances is there required from the government a 'gesture' to restore confidence which may include the mass slaughter of perfectly healthy animals, as well as a huge financial compensation? As Simon Jenkin put it in *The Times*, 'Like some primitive tribe, are we expected to immolate our property to propitiate the raging gods?'—My answer is yes, you are.

The key point of Bikchandani, Hirshleifer and Welch's paper is that since a cascade can be shattered by even a minor public information release, further releases of public information ensure that eventually the society settles into the correct cascade. So suppression of public information, although understandable as an attempt to maintain the current cascade, is in the long-run counter-productive.

Other questions related to the British government's actions include:

Why did the government never implement the proposal by its BSE scientific committee in June 1989 that brains of cattle sent for slaughter should be routinely monitored to check the extent of unrecognized infection?

Why was the ban on 'specified cattle offal', such as brains and spinal columns, for human consumption not introduced until 1989, three years after BSE was discovered?

Why was the ban on use of animal wastes in feed for pigs and poultry not declared until March 1996?

Lesson for Australia

The general lesson to draw from this episode is that public trust in government and scientific advice is fragile. It seems to me that the best way to bolster or maintain public trust in government and scientific advice is to establish or maintain institutional arrangements for the regular dissemination of information generated in the public sector. Moreover this information should be released in a manner that precludes and is seen to preclude manipulation by members of the government, its advisers or the public service.

More specifically in the context of Australia's own beef industries concerns should be felt for the current debate about moves to shift more responsibility for meat inspection away from government and into the hands of the industry itself. The gains from cheating on a system are reaped by the perpetrator but the risk of loss of confidence in the industry and its product is suffered by whole industry. Public confidence in Australian beef, both domestic and international, is a valuable but fragile asset. For any policy change that may threaten such confidence, a careful examination should be conducted to ensure that the potential gains from such a policy change outweigh the costs of any risk to undermining the confidence that the policy may introduce.

NOTES

[1] 'Characterizing Perceived Risk', in *Perilous Progress: Managing the Hazards of Technology* edited by C. Hohenemser, R. Kates, and J. Kasperson, Westview Press, 1985.

[2] See A. V. Banerjee, 'Simple Model of Herd Behavior', *Quarterly Journal of Economics*, 107(3), August 1992, pp. 797-817; S. Bikhchandani, D. Hirshleifer & I. Welch, 'A Theory of Fads, Fashion, Custom, and Cultural Change as Informational Cascades', *Journal of Political Economy*, 100(5), October 1992, pp. 992–1026.

Part Three

Humanities:
Histories, Pathologies and Poetics

THE ROAST BEEF OF OLD ENGLAND
Harriet Ritvo

One of the striking features of the most recent BSE crisis when it began early in 1996 was the reaction of the British government. Its twin policies of denial and neglect, however energetically pursued, never made things better and sometimes made things worse. In part, this reaction can be attributed to the general political and cultural ambience. A philosophy that defined government as the protector of commercial enterprise rather than of its citizenry meant that official concern with beef industry profits consistently overshadowed official concern with the possible public health implications of BSE, whether to cattle, to people, or to members of other species. The indifference to science, and especially the innumeracy, apparently characteristic of most politicians and many journalists, meant that at a time when information about most aspects of BSE—for example, what caused the disease and how it was transmitted—was inconclusive at best, ministers confidently announced that official measures to combat its spread were based on 'scientific evidence'. This was a black box containing nothing.

In addition to national interest, however inadequately defined, more elusive factors like national pride and national passion shaped British reaction to BSE. Both the intensity and the direction of government responses reflected patriotic sensitivities connected with the product most immediately threatened by BSE. Of course, any significant commodity can serve as a metonymy for the nation that produces it, but beef and beef cattle occupied a particularly powerful emblematic position. Thus their special charisma—the identification of the afflicted nation with its afflicted cattle—determined the behaviour of other groups besides the British government. After their first shocked recoil when the possibility of a link to human disease was officially acknowledged, British consumers resumed eating beef at almost their previous rate (although initially supermarkets had to jumpstart demand by halving prices). This gastronomic conservatism was often both urged and understood in terms of patriotism and loyalty, as well as nutrition and value for money. Non-British responses similarly suggested that the plight of British cattle presented an opportunity to express profounder views about the nation they represented. Thus the stalwart commitment proclaimed by other European governments to defend the health of their citizens against the British bovine menace could seem less absolute when BSE was rumoured in their own herds. And unlike their British counterparts who rallied round their sick cattle by continuing to eat them, continental consumers shunned even their own beef in their desire to avoid British contamination.

The association of Great Britain with livestock in general, and with cattle in particular, dates back at least to the agricultural improvers of the eighteenth century. As the size and beauty of their reconfigured animals glorified their own pre-eminence, so the numbers of their herds contributed to national self-sufficiency, which was strategically vital for an island nation frequently at war. Their less eminent fellow countrymen also basked in the reflected glow, attributing many less quantifiable but equally desirable qualities to their enthusiastic meat consumption.[1] Its potent virtues were repeatedly reiterated. For example, in the same way that 'Carnivorous Animals have more Courage, Muscular Strength and Activity,' so a meat-heavy diet was believed to contribute to British 'energy, ... sense of fitness, ... [and] craving for work. ... The beef of the British soldier has always been regarded as a factor in his valour.'[2] Meat-eating was viewed by observers within the British polity and outside it as an essential component of the national character. Well into the second half of the nineteenth century 'our foreign neighbours' were reported to 'believe that all classes in England, excepting *"La grande aristocratie"*, live upon nothing but half raw roast beef and steaks, plum pudding, and brandy "grogs".'[3]

Visitors from Europe also noted with astonishment the amount of flesh regularly eaten in those British households able to afford it.[4] Abundant meat was considered not a luxury of domestic economy, as it might be in less fortunate or carnivorous lands, but a necessity. The sample weekly budgets included in early nineteenth-century editions of Mrs. Rundell's *System of Practical Domestic Economy* assumed that even families of rather modest means would provide each member with more than half a pound of meat each day; several decades later a cookbook writer estimated that every resident of London consumed one hundred and seven pounds of butcher's meat per year, far outstripping the eighty-five pounds consumed by the average Parisian.[5] When asked by her mistress what she and 'her father and brothers ate as a rule for dinner', a Victorian maid replied, 'Why beef and mutton, ma'am, every day! Working people *want* their meat.'[6] William Cobbett warned of the dire consequences of its absence in the poorest households, claiming that *'Meat in the House* is a great source of *harmony*, a great preventer of the temptation to commit those things, which, from small beginnings, lead, finally, to the most fatal and atrocious results'.[7]

Cobbett saw salvation for the needy mainly in terms of bacon, 'a coarse and heavy, but nutritive food,' which, in the view of many dietary experts, was 'only fit to be taken in considerable quantities by robust labouring people.'[8] The iconic meat of the British, however, was beef.[9] As the *Quarterly Journal of Agriculture* complacently noted in 1830, 'our domestic cattle ... [are] the most varied and remarkable in the world, and have long yielded us ... good beef (of which the very name is almost identified with the character and propensities of the nation).'[10] So firm was this association—and so inextricably intertwined was the rhetoric of beefeating with that of patriotism—that the unwary might be led to mistake the metaphor for the fact: thus *Punch* reported that 'a foreign Nobleman ... was horror-struck at being invited to be present at the roasting of a "Baron"'.[11] According to *Household Words*, 'beef is a great connecting link and bond of better feeling between the great classes of the commonwealth', inspiring respect second only to 'the Habeas Corpus and the Freedom of the Press'.[12] As it symbolized the common predilections and loyalties of Britons, so beef emphasized the irreducible alterity of alien cultures. However strikingly they might differ from each other, they were united in their inability to provide this essential sustenance. Thus, 'on the Continent ... tasteless pieces of beef which have been used to make the bouillon are invariably served with sauces ... and the *bifsteak*, so called in honour of the famous English dish, is often a piece of very coarse buffalo'; while 'John Bull in India ... sighs for a Southdown saddle [of mutton] or a Scotch sirloin, and is apt to turn away sorrowfully from the meagre travesty of a joint which, after much trouble, the sharer of his joys and sorrows contrives to place before him'.[13]

Naturalists and agricultural experts, chefs and gourmets agreed that Britain was pre-eminent for the quality of the meat it produced, as well as the quantity it consumed. This additional superiority confirmed the binary distinction between the British and peoples apparently less cathected to animal flesh. Discussions of the national livestock inevitably reiterated a conventional litany of celebration. For example, this consensus asserted that British cattle were 'considered preferable to the cattle of any other country in the world'; that 'the cattle and sheep of this country we may justly regard ... as unequalled in any other territory'; and that 'no country produces finer sheep than Great Britain'.[14] Even a cookbook whose irreverent author disparaged the finished products of British cuisine acknowledged that its raw materials were unrivalled: 'In this country we have the best of all descriptions of butcher's meat in the world, and, with a few exceptions, the worst cooks. If the poor, half-fed meats of France, were dressed as our cooks, for the most part, dress our well-fed excellent meats, they would be absolutely uneatable.'[15]

The virtues of meat could benefit the ailing as well as enhance the vigour of the healthy. It was widely acknowledged that, as a Victorian cookbook for convalescents put it, 'animal food satisfied hunger more completely and for a longer time than vegetables', and that beef and mutton were the most nutritious of meats. Such endorsements often carried some suggestion of moderation, a recognition that, taken in excessive quantity these 'noble viands ... of heroic proportions' offered denser sustenance than 'our modern civilized life' required, even as led by Royal Beefeaters.[16] Or they warned of the intellectual consequences of overindulgence: 'whoever would keep his mind acute and penetrating, should rather exceed on the side of vegetable food.'[17] But the possibilities, however remote and manageable, of indigestion and stupefaction were not universally admitted. The most enthusiastic meat advocates claimed that it was more easily digestable than lighter foods. The late Victorian patients who followed the regimen of the American physician James Salisbury regained their strength on a diet that, in its strictest form, included only egg whites, and black tea or coffee, and the eponymous Salisbury steak. As they recovered they were allowed to relax their regimen somewhat, adding chicken or lamb or even rice, but 'only [as] a relish ... the steak to be four-fifths of the meal'. Patients were assured that once they embraced this diet, they would begin to crave wholesome meat as they had once craved unwholesome vegetables.[18] And some people attributed to carnivory still more surprising efficacy. For example, in 1860 *The Lancet* suggested that meat-eaters had lighter, clearer complexions and that, therefore, 'under a well-devised animal diet it might be possible ... to whiten the blackamoor by feeding, though not by washing'.[19]

If meat-eating in general distinguished Britons from foreigners, it also provided occasions for reinforcing intranational categorizations. The superior sophistication of the metropolis, for example, distinguished its butchers as well as the purveyors of fashionable luxury goods. A late Victorian food critic thus claimed that 'beefsteak ... is only to be had in perfection in London, for it would seem as though country butchers had not learnt the secret of the proper cut'.[20] Even in its unsegmented state, meat also reflected essential social divisions, some elevated kinds 'fit for fine Complexions, idle Citizens,' others, like bacon, 'gross, tough and hard, agreeing chiefly to Country Persons and Hard Labourers.'[21] The hierarchy of class privilege expressed through access to furred and feathered game was echoed in cookbooks. Sometimes elite status was said to confer special nutritional qualities, so that, for example, venison, grouse, pheasant, and, indeed, 'all game' were credited with a 'looseness of texture' that made them 'more digestible' than the flesh of domesticated birds and mammals.[22] Or the dichotomy was embodied in recipes, with venison, hares, rabbits, and game birds grouped for culinary treatment that emphasized their shared distinction from domesticated birds and livestock.[23] Instructions for the commercial production of 'game pie' treated all the creatures that fell under that rubric as interchangeable: 'cut up the game into joints or pieces, and put into a pie dish.'[24] So strong were the associations between social prestige and game, and between game and its conventional preparations, that people who could not aspire to the real thing sometimes borrowed the recipes, metaleptically serving marinated beef in the guise of venison.[25]

More widely available meats were ranked not only by species, but also according to other categories significant in a human context. When it came to ingestion, standard hierarchies of age and sex were inverted. The flesh of mature animals was coarser and tougher than that of delicate young ones, and their fat was less evenly distributed through their muscles. In addition, they had spent more time under what one physician described as 'the very extraordinary ... influence of the genital organs.' Although he believed that even the ovaries impaired 'the flavour of the female', the testicles were the main culprits: 'every day the testes are permitted to remain ... injures the delicacy of the veal of the bull-calf.'[26] Thus experts in domestic economy generally recommended that 'heifer and ox beef are both excellent', and that both were preferable to cow beef, as 'a leg of wether mutton is more desirable than a ewe one'.[27] Indeed, one Victorian commentator forcefully objected to butchering 'the females of ... domesticated mammalia' on 'the joint grounds of impropriety and unwholesomeness', but the meat of cows nevertheless ranked considerably higher than that of bulls, since 'females are sweeter, moister, and easier to be concocted.'[28]

In general, the meat of mature male animals was abominated. Bull beef was easily recognized for its 'strong, unpleasant smell'; and 'ram mutton has a strong, and ... exceedingly disagreeable flavour.'[29] Hearsay evidence suggested that the opposition of delectable females and unpalatable males similarly occurred in some rarely eaten wild creatures; thus, according to Thomas Bewick, among 'Sea-Bears' (a kind of seal) 'the fat and flesh of the old males are very nauseous; but those of the females and the young ... are said to be as good as ... a sucking Pig.'[30] A mid-Victorian agricultural encyclopedia attributed the 'sanguineous odour and flavour' of rams and bulls to masculine behaviour as well as masculine essence, being 'aggravated by ... the exercise of the procreative faculties'.[31] Among livestock, only pigs—the occupants of liminal positions in many taxonomies—broke the gender pattern: 'the flesh of the sow is strong', while 'the flesh of the male ... [makes] the best pork'.[32]

The terms routinely employed to characterize masculine and feminine flesh, and to differentiate males in full exercise of their powers from their neutered brothers, recalled the stereotypical language associated with men and women. The aversion to viewing dominant bulls and rams—the leaders of herds and the fathers of families—as mere table fare may have derived as much from political as from culinary predilections. After all, the strong flavour that made male beef and mutton inappropriate for quotidian consumption seemed not only tolerable but desirable when eating was charged with the special symbolism of preeminence or domination. Thus game, emblematic of class privilege, was valued for exactly those qualities that disqualified the flesh of domestic male animals. Hare was superior to rabbit, 'being much more savoury, and of a higher flavour', and 'buck venison is preferred [to that of the doe] as the choicest meat'.[33] As game was cooked in special ways, so it was prepared distinctively by butchers, to enhance its characteristic rankness. Indeed, according to a plain-spoken Victorian cookbook, aficionados of venison were divided between those who 'like it a little gone, and others a good deal. This state of putrescency is called by gourmands *haut gout*, high tasted; we should rather say at once, stinking.'[34] The allegedly wild white cattle of Scotland and northern England bridged the categories of wild and domestic.[35] Despite their resemblance to ordinary farmyard beasts, their beef tended to be served only on ceremonial occasions, after a ritualized hunt. The Earl of Tankerville thus slaughtered a number of Chillingham cattle to celebrate his son's birthday in 1756, and the Victorian owners of the Lyme Park, Cheshire herd shot one or two animals each Christmas and forwarded some of the beef to Queen Victoria.[36] Although the flesh of these animals—'dark in colour and very full flavoured'—shared the attributes that made the beef of ordinary bulls unacceptable, it was nevertheless considered 'excellent'.[37]

If the consumption of some kinds of animals was mandatory for Britons, and that of others lent social cachet, many creatures existed beyond the gustatory pale. Indeed, their proscribed number had tended to increase since the less finicky medieval period, when any wild animal or bird could end up in a pot or a pan.[38] Fifteenth-century cookbooks included recipes for whale, seal, crane, and peacock, and the taste for red squirrels only declined among the aristocracy in

Tudor times, when suspicions emerged that the rodents were carrying disease.[39] The flesh of speared otters was not only eaten, but also eaten during Lent and on other 'maigre days, from its supposed resemblance to fish, on which otters almost wholly subsist.'[40] The *Naturalist's Library* volume on cetaceans recorded the opinion of 'Dr Caius, the celebrated founder of the College at Cambridge, ... that a Dolphin ... was ... a worthy present to the Duke of Norfolk, who ... [had it] roasted and eaten with porpoise sauce,' as an example of 'the change of tastes produced by modern refinement'.[41] Those who praised this heightened fastidiousness as progress associated it with social and religious order, as well as more delicate sensibilities. As John Goodsir approvingly instructed his comparative anatomy students at the University of Edinburgh, it was appropriate for civilized people to prefer foods 'which were created for [their] special use—e.g. ox, sheep, goat, wheat, [and] barley.'[42]

But what complacent consensus perceived as increasing refinement could also be reinterpreted by dissenters as foregone opportunity or even waste. The circumscribed animal diet of eighteenth- and nineteenth-century Britain, conducive though it might have been to developing solid national character, was open to criticism on other than vegetarian grounds. Pragmatic carnivores reductively lamented the economic loss resulting from the neglect of readily available sources of nourishment. An eighteenth-century dietary reformer reasoned, 'When I considered how cleanly the Hedge-hog feedeth, namely upon Cow's Milk, ... or upon Fruit and Malt; I saw no reason to discontinue this Meat any longer upon some fantastical Dislike.'[43] In 1885, V. I. Holt similarly began his tract *Why Not Eat Insects?* with the rhetoric of rational persuasion, asking his readers to substitute 'a fair hearing ... an impartial consideration ... and an unbiassed judgment' for 'long-existing and deep-rooted public prejudice'. He assured them that the insects he recommended for consumption (in which category he included 'small mollusks and crustaceans ... for the sake of brevity and convenience') were all 'clean, palatable, wholesome, and decidedly more particular in their feeding than ourselves.'[44] The most systematic Victorian attempt to expand the category of edible animals targeted horses and donkeys. Advocates of hippophagy and onophagy, briefly united in the Society for the Propagation of Horse Flesh as an Article of Food, argued not only that a great deal of meat was being wasted, since dogs and cats could not consume the remains of all the horses who died after lives of toil in British streets, fields, and mines, but also that animals destined for the butchers rather than the knackers would experience less brutal treatment in the final months of their lives.[45]

Even in the cause of kindness, however, the British could not be persuaded to eat horses. Their resistance was acknowledged to have deep, although far from primeval, historical roots. Because the pre-Christian inhabitants of Europe had consumed horsemeat with ritual enthuasiasm, early evangelists banned it as part of the comprehensive suppression of pagan observances.[46] And if the practice had nevertheless intermittently reemerged in less prosperous provinces, it had therefore acquired an additional set of undesirable associations with scarcity and backwardness; in 1617, for example, it was reported with disgust that the 'wild Irish ... will feed upon horses dying of themselves, not only upon small want of flesh, but even for pleasure.'[47] Rationalistic horseflesh advocates assumed that in the impregnably Christian societies of nineteenth-century Europe, the danger of recrudescent paganism would pale before such palpable utilitarian advantages as cheap protein and high resistance (compared with beef, for example) to tubercular infection.[48] In France and Belgium, where such distinguished figures as the naturalist Geoffroy Saint Hilaire leant their support, the campaign succeeded. The first horsemeat butcher shop opened in Paris soon after the gala *banquet hippophagique* held at the Grand Hotel in 1865.[49] But neither the francophone example, nor the similar practices of such other European nations as Germany, Russia, and Denmark, where horseflesh reportedly constituted a 'principle item' in the diets of prisoners, softened the intransigence of British diners.[50]

On the contrary, the foreign associations evoked by the horsemeat campaign were more likely to confirm insular resistance. Nor did willingness to try 'chevaline', as this strange meat was christened, necessarily ensure conversion. When the supposed leaders of fashion, or at least the supposed molders of the opinions and habits of their social inferiors, goodnaturedly agreed to try horseflesh, their subsequent enthusiasm was seldom striking. Thus the guests at a French chevaline banquet were reported merely to have been 'perfectly satisfied', and the horseflesh on which Danish prisoners throve tasted 'like coarse beef, yet by no means unpleasantly,' when served plain, and was 'although far from constituting an agreeable product ... not unpalatable' in soup.[51] In 1887 a veteran gastronome admitted that his dislike of chevaline was based on less concrete considerations than its flavor; on the contrary, he usually 'found the soup and other dishes tasty'. But before beginning to eat he had to 'force down my instinctive reluctance to turn the noble horse into an article of food'.[52]

So strong was this default repulsion that it determined British attitudes toward ingestion of related species, and in circumstances where more depended on willingness to partake than the enhancement of dietary choice. As, earlier in the century, William Burchell forthrightly regretted in recounting his adventures in the African bush, 'I could not ... resist altogether the misleading influence of prejudice and habit; and allowed myself, merely because I viewed the meat as horseflesh, to reject food which was really good and wholesome.' Although he praised the greater rationality of his Hottentot attendants, who ate zebras and quaggas with relish, he apparently communicated to them both the strength of his aversion and its approximate source. Identification with the central tenets of British culture required the renunciation of horsemeat. Thus two Hottentots who accepted baptism soon discovered, notwithstanding their lifelong habit of indulgence, 'that they were unable to eat it; ... that it always created a nausea.'[53]

It was, conversely, one of the defining characteristics of foreigners that they craved strange meat, just as gorging on the flesh of domesticated ungulates stereotyped Britons. Just across the Channel the French relished frogs legs and snails, and in remoter lands still odder tastes further confirmed the transgressive predilections of alien peoples.[54] As Thomas Henry Huxley drily commented after inspecting the fish markets of Rio de Janeiro, 'They must eat queer things'.[55] Sometimes these preferences were catalogued with scientific restraint, as contributions to knowledge about either the eater or the eaten, thus conflating eccentric foreigners with the curious creatures they ate as appropriate objects of scrutiny. For example, when describing a new species of jerboa, Thomas Hardwicke noted in passing that 'a tribe of low

Hindus ... esteem them good and nutritious food'.⁵⁶ In his compendium of natural history, William Bingley routinely included such information as that badger flesh, 'which is somewhat similar in taste to that of the wild dog, is much esteemed in Italy, France, and Germany,' and that 'American Indians frequently eat the *flesh* of the skunk.'⁵⁷ The guide to the national collection of animal products at Bethnal Green specified that 'in some countries the flesh of monkeys is eaten'; that 'the flesh of a few bats is eaten'; and that the flesh of many rodents 'serves for food'.⁵⁸

Less restrained and more revealing responses to foreign eating habits ranged from derision to horror. Among some peoples, 'even the rat, which is generally held in abhorrence, is said to be wholesome and savoury food.'⁵⁹ 'A Beef Eater', the pseudonymous author of a book purporting to exhibit 'the natives of various countries at feeding time', distilled this viewpoint, claiming, for example, that 'animals that in England would be looked on with disgust ... are by the Chinese regarded as delicacies.' The loathsome treats included grubs, earthworms, sphinx moth caterpillars, drowned rats, and, worst of all, domestic dogs and cats.⁶⁰ The consumption of companion animals recurred insistently in accounts of exotic eating habits, as both epitome and extreme. A sporting author thus claimed that the flesh of dogs was 'preferred by the negroes to that of any other animal', which demonstrated their 'unnatural and depraved appetite'.⁶¹ According to Bingley, the regrettable habit was widely dispersed: 'Disgusting as it may appear to us, the *flesh* of the dog is a favourite food in many countries.' Not only was it sold like any other meat in the 'markets of Canton', but it was relished in Greenland, North America, and Africa; in the West Indies, on the other hand, he revealed that 'the negroes frequently eat the *flesh* of cats'.⁶² So conventional was the association of the far east with dog eating that by the late Victorian period 'Chinese Edible Dogs', which resembled inelegant reddish pomeranians, were standard fixtures in the 'foreign dogs' class at dog shows.[63]

The categories of science were sometimes invoked to explain the violent aversion provoked by such practices. It was frequently claimed, for example, that willingness to eat other meateaters constituted the dividing line between civilization and barbarism. According to a late nineteenth-century epicure, 'certain very low caste people of India and other lands are said to go in for feeding upon carnivorous animals such as dogs, cats, rats, foxes, leopards, wolves, jackals, and other nasty "brutes" ... a diet which must be characterized as simply disgusting.'[64] Holt, who recommended only insects that were 'strict vegetarians' for human consumption, noted wryly that 'carnivorous animals ... are held unworthy of the questionable dignity of being edible by civilized man'.[65] Victorian housekeepers were confidently instructed that 'beasts of prey ... are never employed as food ... except among savage tribes, or in cases of necessity.' Diverse reasons were offered for this anathema. The flesh of such animals was 'lean ... tough ... coarse and disagreeable'; herbivores were much more 'wholesome'.[66] Or, the dietary restrictions of the Old Testament prohibited the consumption of pawed carnivores, as, indeed, they did of solid-hoofed horses. Equally authoritative religious strictures, however, seldom interfered with Victorian enjoyment of oysters, ham, hare, and lobsters. And as far as members of the order Carnivora were concerned, if the consumption of otters, under the rubric of flesh or of fish, had gone out of fashion long before the nineteenth century, preserved bear meat was still eaten with pleasure when available.[67]

But, as emerged clearly in formulations that pointedly compared European and exotic practises, the real transgression was a social one, derived from the compact understood to exist between dogs and cats (and horses too) and human beings. By eating these animals 'savages' violated a category properly defined by trust and cooperation.[68] Thus, a domestic encyclopedia lamented that 'the *dog*, the faithful companion and friend of man, ... in many parts of the world ... is considered as good food.'[69]

Such errors could be noted with complacency as well as aversion, as unsurprising if regrettable marks of the inferiority of the people who committed them. It was even suggested that dogs bred for food suffered moral and intellectual degeneration, assuming the same relation to European canines that their masters held to European humans. For example, Charles Darwin claimed that, in comparison to English dogs 'valued ... for their mental qualities and sense ... where the dog is kept solely to serve for food, as in the Polynesian islands and China, it is described as an extremely stupid animal.'[70] When other Europeans committed similar transgressions they came in for similar, if moderated condescension; it was assumed that they had somehow mistaken what they were eating—but perhaps by not looking too closely where substitution could be anticipated. Prospective British travellers were warned that 'hundreds of dogs and cats are annually consumed by the inhabitants of the French capital'; the French were furthermore 'accused of being occasionally given to mistake pussy for puss, and to turn dear little tabbies into jugged hare.'[71] More problematic in terms of the hierarchy thus tacitly created was evidence that people of British heritage occasionally relished domestic pets, and not just in a spirit of scientific inquiry. It was reported, for example, that in 'that cosmopolitan city San Francisco', restaurants served 'bow-wow soup' for twelve cents and 'grimalkin steaks' for a quarter.[72] And equivalent outrages occurred much closer to home. In 1771, for example, a 'young country lad' ate 'a whole cat smothered with onions' at a Cambridge public house, reported in the press as no more or less remarkable than his previous epicurean exploit, which was to devour an eight-pound leg of mutton at a single sitting.[73] Well into the Victorian period cat fanciers unhappily acknowledged that 'in some parts of England cats are not wholly despised as an article of diet.'[74] A notorious ring of cat-eaters operated in West Bromwich, near Birmingham, so efficient in their depredations that 'many persons complain that they cannot keep a favourite a week.'[75]

If consuming non-human members of the domestic circle was bad, eating people was worse. Cannibalism figured ubiquitously as the essence of savagery. So inextricably intertwined were these attributes that the logic associating them frequently operated in reverse: if all cannibals were savages, then all savages were cannibals. As a result, many of the exotic peoples encountered by British explorers and colonizers were tarred, at least tentatively, with this brush. Fijians were alleged to butcher and bake the extremities before putting their victim to death; indeed he might be offered a final meal of 'his own cooked flesh'. One chief was reported to have eaten nine hundred people.[76] The anthropophagy of the indigenous New Zealanders was endlessly rehearsed, its abandonment a triumph of the imperial mission. The same earthen ovens in which, at the end of the nineteenth century, they cooked potatoes thus 'probably, in cannibal times ... also served for the *long pig* in which they delighted.'[77] The Tahitians, too, had been reclaimed by 'the humanizing influence of British exertions' from their original position 'amongst the most degraded of the human race', practicing 'cannibalism and the most barbarous rites'.[78] The book of anthropological queries promulgated by the British Association in 1874 to guide 'travellers and residents in uncivilized lands' contained a whole section on 'Cannibalism', immediately after that on 'Food'. The first question asked, relatively innocuously, 'Does cannibalism prevail?' but the second exposed underlying assumptions: 'If it no longer prevails, are there any traditions as to its once having been known?'[79]

Cannibalism was reprehended in aversive language even stronger than that applied to pet-eating. 'Habitual and systematic' cannibalism was 'the most extraordinary and ... revolting eating custom'.[80] Indulgence in human flesh could even jeopardize membership in the human race. *Punch* compared 'the Manyeuma people' unfavorably with the vegetarian gorillas who lived near them: 'Is cannibalism ... the outcome of a higher degree ... in the scale of development—a stage more distinctly human?'[81] The motivations most frequently proposed for this behaviour made it seem still worse. Hunger was generally dismissed as a possibility, or displaced into the remote past.[82] In 1873, for example, *Nature* reported that the 'otherwise gentle Monbuttas' were 'habitual cannibals', although they lived among plentiful herds of 'elephants, buffaloes, antelopes, and wild swine.'[83] Savages thus ate their neighbors and their enemies not to assuage basic needs, which would have been understandable, if not necessarily excusable, but to indulge gratuitous viciousness. In 1831, the London Phrenological Society heard that 'in New Zealanders, and other Savage nations ... the custom did not proceed from hunger, but for the gratification of the revengeful passions.'[84] So clearly axiomatic was the low rank of cannibals on the scale of human civilization, that even the fact that some cultures reprobated in this way possessed more elevated attributes, including belief in a single deity, was sometimes recorded as cause for puzzlement, but not as reason to reconsider either the implications or the existence of anthropophagy.[85]

As in all taxonomies, however, the meaning of the categories was not essential or intrinsic. If cannibalism confirmed the barbarity of exotic peoples, it had no such implications when committed by people incontestably civilized. On the basis of hard evidence, the only people who indisputably qualified as habitual cannibals were of European stock. Travellers who sailed the high seas were liable to shipwreck, and until well into the nineteenth century it was assumed that *in extremis* surviving mariners would kill and eat each other.[86] Explorers marooned in terrestrial wastes, such as members of the Franklin expedition that disappeared in quest of the Northwest Passage in 1845, routinely made similarly pragmatic calculations.[87] The extent to which such behaviour had been regarded as normal and justifiable not only by sailors, but by Britons in general, became obvious in 1884, when Captain Tom Dudley and Mate Edwin Stephens of the yacht *Mignonette*, who had been rescued after suffering shipwreck and extreme subsequent exposure, received the death sentence for the murder of one of their shipmates. Their arrest and prosecution greatly surprised the accused malefactors, who had voluntarily told the whole story, killing included, when they had arrived home. The conviction outraged much of the public, more inclined to treat the brave survivors as heroes than as criminals, so that when Queen Victoria ultimately pardoned them, *The Times* complained of the 'mawkish sympathy' they received.[88] The case of *Regina v. Dudley and Stephens* thus marked the beginning of a new legal era, giving notice that, no matter how extenuating their circumstances, future cannibals could no longer assume that British polity was on their side. But, although the decision provoked a great deal of commentary, it was nowhere hailed as marking the emergence of the nation from an existing condition of barbarism.

Even less exigent cannibalism, if it occurred on home ground, was condemned in terms that seemed relatively mild. When cannibalism was announced at Saint Thomas's Hospital, *The Lancet* reported with relief that the youth who had 'cooked and eaten a small piece of human flesh' taken from a corpse was an assistant in the chemical laboratory, rather than one of the medical students, 'who are gentlemen by birth and education'. But even though he did not belong to this elite group, the erring assistant was not therefore classified among the ranks of savages. He lost his job, but his behaviour was otherwise castigated merely as 'foolish and indecent'.[89] And his eccentric dining habits brought no more generalized disgrace upon his fellow citizens than did that of the cat-eaters of West Bromwich. In a nation self-defined as quintessentially civilized, such lapses inevitably appeared as regrettable eccentricities rather than representative sins. No matter how many people they ate, the British were never classified as *Homo europaeus anthropophagus*. As one anti-vegetarian had concretely and complacently put it, 'those who inhabit the country of roast beef are ... little in danger of seeing the limbs of their friends exposed to sale in their markets'.[90] It has turned out, however, that the noble joint may conceal other hazards. Exactly what they are remains to be seen.

NOTES

[1] The symbolic significance of meat eating, as of other patterns of food consumption and non-consumption, has been analyzed by anthropologists and sociologists concerned with a range of human societies. See, for example, Mary Douglas, Purity and Danger: An analysis of concepts of pollution and taboo (London: Routledge and Kegan Paul, 1966) and 'Deciphering a Meal', in Implicit Meanings: Essays in anthropology (London: Routledge and Kegan Paul, 1975), 249-275; Marcel Détienne and Jean-Pierre Vernant, eds, The Cuisine of Sacrifice Among the Greeks, trans. Paula Wissing (Chicago: University of Chicago Press, 1989); Jack Goody, Cooking, Cuisine and Class: A study in comparative sociology (Cambridge: Cambridge University Press, 1982); Julia Twigg, 'Vegetarianism and the Meanings of Meat', in Anne Marcott, ed., The Sociology of Food and Eating: Essays on the sociological significance of food (Aldershot, Hants.: Gower, 1983), 18-30; and Nick Fiddes, Meat: A natural symbol (London: Routledge, 1991).

[2] John Arbuthnot, An Essay Concerning the Nature of Aliments, and the Choice of Them, According to the Different Constitutions of Human Bodies (London: J. Tonson, 1732), 225; J. Milner Fothergill, The Food We Eat: Why we eat it and whence it comes (London: Griffith and Farran, 1882), 53-54.

[3] Tabitha Tickletooth [Charles Selby], The Dinner Question: or, how to dine well and economically (London: Routledge, Warne, and Routledge, 1860), 37.

[4] C. Anne Wilson, Food and Drink in Britain, from the Stone Age to Recent Times (London: Constable, 1973), 97; Frederick William Hackwood, Good Cheer: The romance of food and feasting (New York: Sturgis and Walton, 1911), 172, 304.

[5] John Burnett, Plenty and Want: A social history of diet in England from 1815 to the present day (London: Methuen, 1983), 64, 88; Hints for the Table: or the economy of good living (London: George Routledge and Sons, 1866), 58.

[6] Eleanor E. Orlebar, Food for the People; or, lentils and other vegetable cookery (London: Sampson, Low, Marston, Searle and Rivington, 1879), 16.

7 William Cobbett, Cottage Economy (London: C. Clement, 1822), 162. During the early nineteenth century, many of the rural and urban poor went largely without meat, although well-paid industrial workers could eat meat every day. Betty McNamee, 'Trends in Meat Consumption', in T. C. Barker, J. C. McKenzie, and John Yudkin, eds, Our Changing Fare: Two hundred years of British food habits (London: MacGibbon and Kee, 1966), 76-79.

8 J. S. Forsyth, The Natural and Medical Dieteticon: or, practical rules for eating, drinking, and preserving health, on principles of easy digestion (London: Sherwood, Jones, 1824), 236.

9 For a representative formulation of this mythic affinity, see Maguelonne Toussaint-Samat, History of Food, trans. Anthea Bell (Cambridge, MA: Blackwell, 1992), 103.

10 'On the Origin and Natural History of the Domestic Ox, and its Allied Species', Quarterly Journal of Agriculture 2 (1830), 196-197.

11 'O! the Roast Beef', Punch 68 (January 16, 1875), 31.

12 Quoted in Peter Lund Simmonds, The Curiosities of Food: or, the dainties and delicacies of different nations obtained from the animal kingdom (London: R. Bentley, 1859), 2-3.

13 Anne Walbank Buckland, Our Viands: Whence they come and how they are cooked, with a bundle of old recipes from cookery books of the last century (London: Ward and Downey, 1893), 75; Arthur Robert Kenney-Herbert, Culinary Jottings for Madras, or, A Treatise in Thirty Chapters on Reformed Cookery for Anglo-Indian Exiles, ed. Leslie Forbes (1885; rpt. Prospect Books: Totnes, Devon, 1994), 102-103.

14 William Bingley, Useful Knowledge; or a familiar account of the various productions of nature, mineral, vegetable, and animal, which are chiefly employed for the use of man (London: Baldwin and Craddock, 1831), III, 94; Duncan MacDonald, Cattle, Sheep, and Deer (London: Steele and Jones, 1872), 8; Duncan McDonald, The New London Family Cook; or, Town and Country Housekeeper's Guide (London: Albion Press, 1808), 25.

15 The Guide to Service: The cook (London: Charles Knight, 1842), 12-13.

[16] Edmund S. and Ellen J. Delamere, Wholesome Fare or the Doctor and the Cook: A manual of the laws of food and the practice of cookery (London: Lockwood, 1868), 3, 341-342.

[17] J. S. Forsyth, The Natural and Medical Dieteticon, 75.

[18] Anna K. Eccles, A Manual of What to Eat and How to Cook It for Salisbury Patients (New York: Kellogg, 1897), 15, 63-64.

[19] 'Feeding the Negro White', The Lancet, June 2, 1860, 555.

[20] Buckland, Our Viands, 75.

[21] Thomas Moffett, Health's Improvement: or, rules comprizing and discovering the nature, method and manner of preparing all sorts of foods used in this nation (London: T. Osborne, 1746), 103.

[22] Hints for the Table: or, the economy of good living (London: George Routledge and Sons, 1866), 7.

[23] See, for example, The Guide to Service: The cook, 38.

[24] Douglas's Encyclopædia. Second Edition (London: William Douglas and Sons, n.d.[ca. 1910]), 289.

[25] Wilson, Food and Drink in Britain, 109.

[26] J. A. Paris, Treatise on Diet: With a view to establish, on practical grounds, a system of rules for the prevention and cure of the diseases incident to a disordered state of the digestive functions (London: Sherwood, Gilbert and Piper, 1837), 187-188.

[27] Mary Barrett Brown, Fish, Flesh and Fowl: When in season, how to select, cook, and serve (London: L. Upcott Gill, 1897), 46; R. W. Dickson, A Complete System of Improved Live Stock and Cattle Management (London: Thomas Kelly, 1824), I, 28.

[28] Robert Mudie, Domesticated Animals, Popularly Considered, in their Structure, Habits, Localities, Distribution, Natural Relations, and Influence upon the Progress of Human Society (Winchester: D. E. Gilmour, 1839), 241-242; Moffett, Health's Improvement, 126.

[29] Brown, Fish, Flesh and Fowl, 46; The Guide to Service: The cook, 229.

[30] Thomas Bewick, A General History of Quadrupeds (Newcastle-upon-Tyne: T. Bewick and Son, 1824), 512.

[31] William Ewart, 'Meat', in John C. Morton, ed., A Cyclopedia of Agriculture, Practical and Scientific (Glasgow: Blackie and Son, 1855), II, 396.

[32] Thomas Webster and Mrs. Parkes, An Encyclopedia of Domestic Economy (London: Longman, Brown, Green, and Longman, 1847), 375.

[33] Webster and Parkes, Encyclopedia of Domestic Economy, 377, 379.

[34] The Guide to Service: The cook, 230.

[35] See Harriet Ritvo, 'Race, Breed, and Myths of Origin: Chillingham cattle as ancient Britons', Representations 39 (1992), 1-22.

[36] Frank Graham, Wooler, Ford, Chillingham and the Cheviots (Newcastle: Frank Graham, 1976), 30; Charles Oldham, 'The Lyme Park Herd of Wild White Cattle', Zoologist 15 (1891), 85.

[37] Charles G. Barrett, 'The Wild Cattle at Chillingham', Transactions of the Norfolk and Norwich Naturalists Society (1875), 54; Laisters F. Lort, 'The White Cattle of Vaynol Park', Transactions of the North Staffordshire Field Club 33 (1898-1899), 56.

[38] Jack C. Drummond and Anne Wilbraham, The Englishman's Food: A history of five centuries of English diet (London: Jonathan Cape, 1939), 119.

[39] Maxime McKendry, Seven Hundred Years of English Cooking, ed. Arabella Boxer (London: Treasure Press, 1973), 14; Wilson, Food and Drink in Britain, 83-84.

[40] Bingley, Useful Knowledge, III, 48.

[41] Robert Hamilton, The Natural History of the Ordinary Cetacea or Whales (Edinburgh: W. H. Lizars, 1837), 243.

[42] John Goodsir, 'Lectures on Comparative Anatomy', student notes, Summer Session, 1858 (Lecture 2, May 20th), Edinburgh University Library Special Collections Gen 580D-581D.

[43] Moffett, Health's Improvement, 158.

[44] Vincent M. Holt, Why Not Eat Insects? (1885; rpt. London: British Museum (Natural History), 1988), 3, 4, 9-10.

45 F.J. Simoons, Eat Not This Flesh: Food avoidances in the old world (Madison: University of Wisconsin Press, 1961), 85.

46 W. W. Cazalet, 'Hippophagy and Onophagy', Temple Bar 19 (1866), 31-32; Jean-Pierre Digard, L'homme et les animaux domestiques: Anthropologie d'une passion (Paris: Fayard, 1990), 72-73.

47 Simoons, Eat Not This Flesh, 84; quoted in Wilson, Food and Drink in Britain, 76.

48 Toussaint-Samat, History of Food, 98.

49 Simoons, Eat Not This Flesh, 85; Cazalet, 'Hippophagy and Onophagy', 33-34.

50 'Horse-flesh as Food for Man', The Lancet, October 31, 1857, 457.

51 Cazalet, 'Hippophagy and Onophagy', 34; 'Horse-flesh as Food for Man', 457.

52 An Old Bohemian, Dishes and Drinks; or, philosophy in the Kitchen (London: Ward and Downey, 1887), 52-53.

53 William Burchell, Travels in the Interior of Southern Africa (London: Longman, Hurst, Rees, Orme, and Brown, 1822, 1824), II, 83, 238.

54 See Goody, Cooking, Cuisine and Class, 146.

55 Quoted in Adrian Desmond, Huxley: The devil's disciple (London: Michael Joseph, 1994), 58.

56 Thomas Hardwicke, 'Description of a Species of Jerboa, found in the upper Provinces of Hindustan ... ', Linnean Society of London. Transactions 8 (1804), 281.

57 Bingley, Useful Knowledge, III, 53-54, 40.

58 Peter Lund Simmonds, Animal Products: Their preparation, commerical uses, and value (New York: Scribner, Welford, and Armstrong: 1877), 1, 2.

59 Webster and Parkes, Encyclopedia of Domestic Economy, 380.

60 A Beef Eater, Illustrations of Eating: Displaying the omnivorous character of man; and exhibiting the natives of various countries at feeding time (London: John Russell Smith, 1847), 36-37.

[61] W. Taplin, The Sportsman's Cabinet (London, 1803), I, 14.

[62] Bingley, Useful Knowledge, III, 24-25, 38.

[63] Hugh Dalziel, British Dogs: Their varieties, history, characteristics, breeding, management, and exhibition (London: 'The Bazaar', 1881), 447.

[64] An Old Bohemian, Dishes and Drinks, 54.

[65] Holt, Why Not Eat Insects?, 11.

[66] Webster and Parkes, Encyclopedia of Domestic Economy, 371.

[67] Cazalet, 'Hippophagy and Onophagy', 35; Frederick Markham, Shooting in the Himalayas. A journal of sporting adventures and travel in Chinese Tartary, Ladac, Thibet, Cashmere (London: Richard Bentley, 1854), 145.

[68] Simoons, Eat Not This Flesh, 104.

[69] Webster and Parkes, Encyclopedia of Domestic Economy, 380.

[70] Charles Darwin, The Variation of Animals and Plants under Domestication (New York: D. Appleton, 1892), II, 205.

[71] Beef Eater, Illustrations of Eating, 38; Old Bohemian, Dishes and Drinks, 55. 'Puss' was a slang term for 'hare'.

[72] Hackwood, Good Cheer, 290.

[73] The British Chronicle, 14 November 1771, quoted in Clifford Morsley, News from the English Countryside, 1750-1850 (London: Harrap, 1979), 71-72.

[74] Gordon Stables, Dogs in Their Relation to the Public (Social, Sanitary and Legal) (London: Cassell, Petter, and Galpin, 1877), 14-15.

[75] 'Eating Cats at West Bromwich', Live Stock Journal and Fancier's Gazette 2 (1875), 756.

[76] Thomas Williams, quoted in George Stocking, Victorian Anthropology (New York: Free Press, 1987), 90.

[77] Buckland, Our Viands, 9.

[78] W. Linnaeus Martin, A General Introduction to the Natural History of Mammiferous Animals, with a Particular View of the Physical History of Man (London: Wright, 1841), 267.

[79] British Association for the Advancement of Science, Notes and Queries on Anthropology for the Use of Travellers and Residents in Uncivilized Lands (London: Edward Stanford, 1874), 45.

[80] Beef Eater, Illustrations of Eating, 40.

[81] 'Gorillas and Ghouls', Punch 68 (January 16, 1875), 31.

[82] See, for example, Nature 35 (1887), 350 (untitled note).

[83] 'Scientific Serials', Nature 8 (1873), 375.

[84] 'London Phrenological Society', The Lancet (1832), 488.

[85] For example, the Monbuttas 'ranked as one of the most important monarchical states of Central Africa ... [and] recognized one supreme being'. The Battas of Sumatra were 'so far advanced in civilization' that they 'actually have laws to regulate the eating of criminals and prisoners of war'; according to Sir Stamford Raffles they too 'acknowledged a Supreme Being'. 'Scientific Serials', 375; Beef Eater, Illustrations of Eating, 40; Hackwood, Good Cheer, 339.

[86] For instances of eighteenth- and nineteenth-century maritime cannibalism, see A. W. Brian Simpson, Cannibalism and the Common Law: The story of the tragic last voyage of the Mignonette and the strange legal proceedings to which it gave rise (Chicago: University of Chicago Press, 1984), 114-143.

[87] See Simpson, Cannibalism and the Common Law, 147-160 for land expeditions similarly driven to cannibalism.

[88] Simpson, Cannibalism and the Common Law, 10-11, 89, 248-250.

[89] 'Cannibalism', The Lancet (September 21, 1867), 373.

[90] [Brougham], 'Ritson on Abstinence from Vegetable Food', 133.

KURU:
THE PURSUIT OF THE PRIZE AND THE CURE[1]

Hank Nelson

Reports of the scientific investigation of the disease, kuru, that afflicted people in New Guinea have recently appeared in the international media.[2] Two events have turned attention to what to most commentators is an exotic disease, an exotic location and a distant time: the hysteria over Mad Cow Disease and the charging of Daniel Carleton Gajdusek, Nobel prize winner, with the sexual abuse of a youth. A major advance in understanding presenile dementias and in the career of Gajdusek had their beginnings in New Guinea in 1957. The reports arising from the coincidence of attention on the research and the researcher have been marred by many errors of fact, tangled chronologies and doubtful generalizations. In the most simplistic reports the scientists seem to arrive suddenly among villagers with no previous contact with the outside world, and the practical and moral complexities of the research are ignored. This is an attempt to locate the research, not in the exotic, but in a particular time and place, offer a perception of some of the individuals and groups involved, and outline a few events with a significance beyond the moment of their happening.

People, parts of people, evidence and arguments came and went, but kuru began, flourished and declined in one place, the Okapa area of the Eastern Highlands of Papua New Guinea. It is an area about fifty kilometres across, home of thirty-five thousand people spread through some one hundred and sixty villages.

In 1956 and 1957 when the doctors and sufferers first came together in the villages, Okapa was a patrol post in the Australian Territory of New Guinea, held under the 1946 United Nations trusteeship agreement. The Australian Territories of Papua and New Guinea had one unified administration with its capital in Port Moresby but the Australians agreed to keep the status of New Guinea and its statistics separate from those of Papua so that there could be regular auditing of their stewardship.[3] The people of Okapa, and of all the Trust Territory of New Guinea, had no nation, and so no nationality: in 1957 they were Australian Protected Persons.

In 1957 nearly a quarter of Papua and New Guinea was not under full government control, all of it in the central highlands or on the highland fringe.[4] Over a quarter of a million people out of a total population of 1.7 million were thought to live in the lands sometimes influenced, but not governed, by the Australians. Just three Papua New Guineans were nominated, and none were elected, to sit in the Legislative Council that met in Port Moresby. For most people, and all people in the highlands, 'government' was one or two Australians, half a dozen Papua New Guinean policemen carrying .303 rifles, and a line of carriers.[5] Five times during that year Papua New Guineans attacked patrols, but in only one case was anyone killed. Not one of the Papua New Guinean policeman on patrol was an officer, and it was accepted that it would be 'some considerable time before suitably qualified persons are available'.[6]

In 1957 the Territory Department of Public Health spent twice that of any of the other big departments: District Services, Education, and Agriculture.[7] Education, the obvious competitor for money for social good, had been slow to spend in the postwar: only about one hundred and fifty Papua New Guineans had reached fourth year in government and mission high schools by 1957, and a few more were on scholarships at Australian secondary schools.[8] Health had been able to plan, recruit and spend more effectively than other departments because all Australians who wanted to do good in the Territory agreed that they should improve the health of Papua New Guineans, because senior officials across departments recognized the enormity of the postwar health problem, and because Dr John Gunther was appointed Director of the Department of Public Health. Gunther arrived in Port Moresby in 1946, the first postwar Director, and in 1957 he was appointed Assistant Administrator to Donald Cleland. He was seen as likely at some time to be appointed Administrator. Gunther, born in 1910, graduated in medicine from Sydney in 1935, and worked in the Solomon Islands and Mount Isa before serving in the RAAF as a malariologist. At the end of the war he was a Squadron Leader commanding a unit doing research into scrub typhus in the New Guinea islands. He inherited a department with five doctors and an office with a dirt floor and the top half of the walls made of chicken wire.

Gunther was often aggressive, carrying himself like the boxer he had been in his university days; he was energetic; and he had the capacity to see the main problem, decide on a practical and sometimes unorthodox solution, and pursue it vigorously. To get basic health care into the villages he trained Native Medical Assistants who could be illiterate, and who might make mistakes, but who on balance would quickly bring known effective treatment to communities that could not otherwise be reached. Having failed to obtain doctors in Australia and Great Britain, Gunther persuaded the Australian government to release refugee doctors in Australia from their two-year work contracts and allow them to practise medicine in Papua and New Guinea. After a three months' course at the Australian School of Pacific Administration in Sydney, refugee doctors arrived in Port Moresby in 1950. 'Some were', Gunther said, 'first rate, a few were misfits, the majority were good industrious public servants'. Of the sixty-seven doctors in the Department of Public Health in 1957 most were East European via Australian migrant camps: they were 'the backbone of the service'.[9] Another five Hungarian doctors arrived in that year, a result of the most recent upheaval in Eastern Europe.[10]

Measured by the numbers of deaths of hospital patients, pneumonia, malaria and tuberculosis were the main diseases threatening the lives of Papua New Guineans. On patrols medical officers most frequently treated skin diseases, tropical ulcers and yaws, the conditions that so often meant that villagers were disfigured with scabs, scales and weeping sores, nearly all of which responded quickly to penicillin or other 'shoots' (injections). But there were other significant problems, many of them outside the experience of most medical practitioners in Australia—or Eastern Europe. There were some two thousand people in Leper or Hansenide colonies,[11] and the first government leprologist was appointed in 1956. Australian officials were uncertain how many infants died, or why they died, but they knew that thousands of lives could be saved every year if children under three could be protected against respiratory infections, diarrhoea and gastro-enteritis.

All this is set down to make the point that the discovery of a new disease with spectacular and intriguing symptoms, progress and distribution was significant, but it was taking place in a Territory where over two hundred thousand were beyond almost all state or mission medical services, where diseases that had slight impact on the eighteen thousand Europeans in the Territory, such as pneumonias, tuberculosis, malaria and dysentery, were killing thousands, and where infant malnutrition and mortality were high. Public health officers could reasonably argue that in a service of just sixty-seven doctors, an influx of funds and specialists directed at mundane and known priorities would save many Melanesian lives. They could not all be expected to share the sense of urgency and importance that some outsiders might put on a new disease.

Many Australian politicians and officials were uncertain about whether or not they owned the Territory of Papua and New Guinea. Papua was certainly theirs; New Guinea was held in trust; and presumably whatever happened to the two territories they would go together. When asked to say what would happen to the Territory Australians said they would let Papua New Guineans decide when they were ready. That set no specific constitutional target, and eliminated no possibility. In their uncertain relationship with Papua New Guinea, Australians were often aggressively possessive. It was, they thought, essential for their defence, although they were just beginning to have doubts about that. It was the one place beyond Australian shores where Australians played a significant role as other than a minor partner in the affairs of the world. They desperately wanted to be better administrators than the old colonial powers—in fact they so wanted to be seen as different they denied parallels with Africa and they would not accept that Papua New Guinea was a colony and Australians in Papua and New Guinea were colonizers.[12] For the moment, Papua and New Guinea was theirs to direct and develop, if not to possess, and it was their frontier—a frontier of adventure and of knowledge that Australians would exploit to the benefit of all and the rest of the world would come to recognize the Australian achievement.

The people at the centre of the story, the people who had the disease, were the Fore. Like most peoples in Papua New Guinea they had no group name for themselves. They were simply the 'one people'.[13] The Fore called the disease kuru, and it meant to shiver or tremble. It is the one word of their language that the Fore have given to the world. And the disease spread into neighbouring peoples on the north and east, the peoples with whom the Fore had most transactions. But it was centred on the South Fore. In 1958, in one of the first censuses in the area, there were seven thousand people in the South Fore. The Fore were Eastern Highlanders by administrative district, by language group, and by other characteristics of their culture.

The Fore are the most eastern of the Eastern Highlanders.[14] Beyond them are other peoples with different languages, different material cultures and different social organization—such as the Anga or Kukukuku on the east. To the south there is uninhabited, rough, ravined, forested country and there the Fore have no immediate neighbours.

They are, then, frontier people, with more land and more forest, and consequently more hunting and collecting, than most highlanders. Before contact they lived in small hamlets behind defensive palisades. One of the refugee doctors, looking at a split log fence, said it reminded him of the palings around his home in the Baltic.[15] Most of the hamlets contained just seventy to one hundred and twenty people. The men lived separately in a men's house, and young boys left their mothers' homes when about seven. Some of the hamlets and gardens were at over seven thousand feet altitude and all houses were probably at over three thousand and five hundred feet—so nights were cold and people crowded about smoky fires in the round log-walled, thatch-roofed houses. The people kept pigs and the basic crop was sweet potatoes, but with a variety of other crops such as taro, yams, sugar cane, pitpit, and bananas.

In 1930 two Australian goldminers, Michael Leahy and Michael Dwyer, and their New Guinean team on their way to the Papuan coast passed to the west of the Fore.[16] They saw the west of Mount Michael, later named after Michael Leahy, and the Fore could see the east of that same massive mountain rising to twelve thousand feet. In the 1930s the Fore heard and watched the first aeroplane fly overhead, and if they did not see Edward (Ted) Ubank, Alexander (Lax) Peadon and the Ashton brothers (Sid and Lea) who were prospecting somewhere in the area, they heard about them. Rumours and physical evidence—such as a piece of cloth—were travelling south.

During the war some Australians escaped south through the edge of the Fore country, and at least three aeroplanes, one of them Japanese, crashed in Fore country.[17] An epidemic of dysentery, probably introduced by the Japanese on the northern edge of the highlands, spread widely, and killed an unknown number of Fore.

Inevitably, all of this had an unsettling effect on the Fore. They had meetings and cults developed as people searched for the protective ritual, or for the ritual that would unlock the new power and wealth that seemed to be just beyond their borders.

The first administration patrol into the Fore in 1947 went to recover a particular western artefact that had entered the area. In 1943 an officer on a wartime patrol to the northeast of the Fore put his rifle down while he 'paid a brief visit to the bush'. Joyo, a visitor from Osena on the borders of the North Fore, grabbed the rifle. Later, through people who lived near Kainantu, Joyo obtained bullets and knowledge. Joyo used the rifle in local warfare, and in September 1947 a bigman of Moife, just north of the Fore, went to meet Don Grove patrolling in the Kamano to tell him that enemies of the Moife and their Fore allies had hired Joyo and his rifle to attack them. Already, a Moife leader and a Kagu woman had been shot.[18] In the history of pacification in Papua and New Guinea this was a rare case of a rifle, the ultimate tool of pacification, moving in advance of the contact frontier.[19]

Ian Skinner, who led the patrol south from Kainantu in October 1947, was ambushed, showered with arrows, and the interpreter's shouted demand for talks was met with the reply 'we like this sort of thing'— and more arrows. Eventually Joyo handed the rifle to an intermediary who brought it in, and Skinner rewarded him with presents. The rifle, Skinner reported, was a .303 in excellent condition and recently used. In the encounter a policeman had been slightly wounded with an arrow, and one or two Fore or their neighbours may have been shot.[20] Further south in the Fore, after the patrol left Ibusa, a group of shield-carrying warriors, trying to take advantage of a distracted enemy, made a sudden raid on the village. Skinner returned, and by firing into soft garden ground in front of the raiders, forced them to flee. Ibusa was burnt, but no-one killed in the raid, and as Skinner alone did the shooting he was confident that none of the raiders had been shot.[21] Elsewhere in the Fore the patrol was greeted by nervous but friendly people. At Kagu and other previously uncontacted villages the people 'lined' to have the census taken. They must have learnt from other villagers that this was what government officers expected, and they behaved accordingly. Skinner thought the people too 'unsettled' to attempt to take a census, and just observed, talked and moved on.

In the four or five years that the Australians were gradually asserting their rule on the Fore, the fight for the rifle was probably the most violent encounter. Skinner predicted that the 'Forei' were ready to accept control, and he was right. Government officers on later patrols adopted what was then standard practice. The exploratory patrols picked up men to be taken back to Kainantu where they could see what the government did and learn some *Tok Pisin*, they told the people to build roads, appointed village officials (*luluais* and *tultuls*), and they set up police posts manned by Papua New Guinean police. Corporal Nalakor and Constables Merakami and Pakau opened the first police post at Moke in January 1951.[22] Nalakor, praised for building the substantial police barracks and rest house on a ridge of the Lamari and Bena River divide, and gaining the confidence of the people, was soon suspended. He shot a Purosa man said to be part of a force attacking Kasaru. Although the investigating officer, G. Linsley, found no evidence of abuse of power, he thought it best to send Nalakor, the best in the police detachment at 'consolidating control amongst new natives', back to Kainantu.[23]

At the same time other patrols coming south and east through Lufa and Henganofi were extending control into the Fore neighbours on the west and north: the Gimi, Keiagana, Yate, and Yagaria. They too established their police posts, collected the ambitious and daring to take back to Goroka, and instructed the people to make roads, bury their dead and stop inter-tribal fighting. The people participated in secular and spiritual ceremonies that acknowledged change. In August 1950 near Tarabo Patrol Officer Arthur Carey gathered old enemies together for 'the rite of breaking weapons', demonstrated the superiority of the .303 over the bow and arrow, and planted 'tanket' (*Taetsia fructicosa*) to mark the boundary between the warring groups.[24] Further north the Lutherans were encouraging the people to display then break their 'sacred flutes'.[25]

Patrols from Kainantu were also passing through the Fore neighbours on the east: the Awa, Auyana and other groups on the Lamari and its tributaries. All the early patrols from Kainantu, Henganofi and Lufa crossed the boundaries of three, four or more language groups. In 1950 there was not so much a frontier line, but a succession of communities from west of Mount Michael to the Lamari all accommodating radical change.

When Gerry Toogood led a patrol through the Fore in April and May of 1950 he had with him as interpreter a Fore youth of about sixteen whom he had recruited on an earlier patrol. Toogood wrote:

> The progress of these people in the few months since my last patrol is amazing, with the few picks and shovels issued on loan from the station to each village excellent graded roads have been constructed, villages cleaned up and re-built, while several hamlets, the inhabitants of which had earlier broken away from their main groups and taken up scattered locations on strategic peaks because of inter-tribal warfare, have returned to their old sites, new villages having been built near the route of the first patrol.[26]

Most of the people who built the roads had never seen a wheeled vehicle, and they walked miles from the South Fore to reach the end of the road to dig, carry stones, and erect log bridges: payment for roadwork was the one way they could get steel tools.[27] From 1953 the Fore sometimes knew when the *kiap* (government officer) was on his way because they heard the roar of the Landrover, and from 1954 they could follow the sound of his motor bike. The noise of the internal combustion engine, that they had heard in the sky in the 1930s, and that presaged change, had come among them.[28]

The first patrol officers found that many Fore went north well into Kamano country to meet them. People from villages not yet visited pleaded with them to come to their hamlets, and 'lavished' them with food on arrival.[29] By 1952 North Fore men had left to find work with goldminers, at the government agricultural station at Aiyura and around Kainantu. Some had failed to get work, and came home without the prestige of material goods and the stories that made them more than 'bush kanakas'.[30] The Fore who left home cut their plaits and changed their dress, and the new fashions were quickly adopted by many who stayed behind.[31] The Fore planted new crops, some exchanged village to village and some grown from seeds distributed by patrols: potatoes, tomatoes, corn, beans and peanuts.[32] Fowls joined pigs and dogs in the hamlets: by June 1952 the 'chook' (chicken) had reached Moke.[33] From 1954 the Berkshire boar held at Okapa station began spreading his genes through the Fore pigs.[34] In 1954 some men made their own decision to walk to Aiyura, get coffee seedlings from the agricultural station, carry them home, and plant them. In 1957 Iagusa village got its first coffee payment: twenty-three shillings.[35] Papua New Guinean Lutheran and Seventh Day Adventist teachers followed the first patrols, and by 1952 some of them were living in the South Fore. From 1950 a white missionary was in charge of the Lutheran station at Tarabo, northwest of the Fore, but among people at the margin of those suffering from kuru.[36] Headmaster Robert Kaul opened the first government school at Okapa in 1957 with one hundred students: ninety-four boys and six girls.[37]

Nagariso, a Native Medical Orderly, accompanied Skinner on the 1947 patrol, and medical orderlies went on most later patrols. The first European Medical Assistant, D.L. Carroll, patrolled through the Fore with Toogood in 1949. By 1952 a Native Medical Orderly was stationed at Moife and he sometimes brought his limited range of cures south into the Fore.[38] The next year a Native Medical Orderly was posted to Moke, and an aid post was planned for Purosa in the far south.[39] Early government officers reported many obvious signs of ill-health in the Fore: neglected wounds, and yaws so advanced that noses and palates were eaten away and the faceless victims were close to death.[40] In June 1952 Patrol Officer, W.J. Kelly, gathered together fifteen people rotting with yaws and told them to walk back to Kainantu with the Native Medical Orderly. Not one of them went to Kainantu: some walking wounded were then prepared to go to patrols seeking help, but they were not yet ready to make a three-day walk through unknown country for uncertain treatment. The next year Acting District Officer, Harry West, 'despatched' about twenty people to the Kainantu hospital—and apparently they went.[41] But even by the end of 1953 when people were themselves choosing to walk to Moke for injections against yaws, the government officers knew that they were not seeing most of the sick with symptoms that did not break the skin.[42] The government officers' belief that better health came with them and followed them helped convince them—and Australians in general—that they were right to intervene in the Fore, and to regret that they could not bring change more quickly.

If government officers thought there was a barrier to their work in the Fore then it was 'rampant' sorcery.[43] The Fore believed that many people were being killed by sorcery, and accusations of sorcery caused disputes that became fights. The government officers recognized one method of killing, *sanguma*, from elsewhere in New Guinea: a victim was usually knocked unconscious, and thin slivers of wood were inserted into various points of the body. The man recovered, went home, and often sickened and died—either because vital organs had been punctured or from infection.[44] At the previously uncontacted village of Yagusa, Kelly saw the small leaf-wrapped bundles of meat used to determine the name of the sorcerer: each parcel was given a name of a possible sorcerer and the least cooked was the guilty man.[45] Soon after he was appointed to Okapa, John McArthur told the people to assemble and 'finish the thing once and for all'. People came forward and handed over their powders, bits and pieces, and the wires that had replaced slivers of wood in *sanguma*. All were publicly burnt, and what would not burn was buried under the posts of the *kiap*'s house. McArthur told the people that he would punish not only those who practised sorcery, but the next man who came to him and made an accusation based on divination.[46] Explanations about a rational world, threats and public denunciations had little effect. John Colman, who replaced McArthur, was soon reporting that sorcery was 'the main impeding factor. ... It is the cause of their fears and suspicions ...'.[47]

Government officers with experience elsewhere in the highlands commented on the speed of the imposition and acceptance of peace in the Fore. McArthur wrote: 'Stockades everywhere are rotting away'.[48] In many areas it came with just two or three patrols, and with no Australian or Papua New Guinean officers resident in the area.

The speed of change was all the more surprising given the violence among precontact Fore. Groups of hamlets, the widest political units with perhaps three hundred people in them, were often at war. When the anthropologists did their detailed genealogies, and they did them often, they found that since 1900 warfare had been the commonest cause of death among men—more frequent than old age or any classification of illness known to the Fore. If what were clearly murders were included then over a quarter of Fore men died violently.[49] Perhaps, it has been said, the Fore welcomed the foreigners as a way to end their own violence. They went to meet the outside world with hope, as well as waiting, disturbed and apprehensive, for it to come to them.

Between 1951 and 1953 the first anthropologists, Ronald and Catherine Berndt, entered the Fore. From their first articles in *Oceania* in 1952 the Fore were known to anthropologists, and known within five years of effective first contact, and almost as soon as they were said to accept the authority of the Australian administration.[50] By 1951 most of the Fore area was declared controlled. In 1953 South Fore was made a separate census division, and at that time nearly three thousand of the South Fore, just less than half of the total, had their names written in village books.[51] In 1954 McArthur built the first permanent government station at Moke, and it was at that time that the government centre officially became Okapa. Already there was a jeep road through to Kainantu: and at Kainantu there was an airstrip and a track to Lae.[52] By 1957 the Fore were at the end of a line connecting them to the rest of the world. Beyond the Fore to the south and east the land was still 'uncontrolled'.[53]

Consider the Fore at about 1957. They had gone through a profound revolution, but much of it had been in their minds—in their non-material culture. In 1920 they could have been confident that they knew as much about the way the world worked as any humans. While they knew communities that spoke differently, dressed differently and organized differently, this was not sufficient to cause the Fore to question the way that they themselves did things. But by 1957 they had encountered rumours, artefacts and people who told them that the world was vastly different from what they had believed, and they had seen that human beings had capacities and could be different in ways unimaginable to them in 1920. They had to accept some changes—like burying their dead, digging pit latrines, making roads and stopping fighting—and some of these changes they welcomed. They also had to change their thinking about their place in the world and their strength and knowledge relative to other peoples. If they wanted equality in this wider world they would have to undergo even more changes than had taken place. They still had their own land and their own language, and nearly all of the time when they were in their own homes and gardens they were dominant. Like many other highlanders they did not seem overwhelmed by the prospect of another revolution.

But the Fore had an affliction that other highlanders, other peoples in the world, did not have. A pestilence had come among them just as they were hearing of, and going through, these profound changes.

In 1950 Arthur Carey, patrolling on the east of the Fore in the Inibi-Kimigomo area was told that sorcery was the cause of several deaths. He described the symptoms of two cases seen at Kauna:

> The temperature of patient however is below normal, about ninety-two, and intense shakings, reminiscent of a heavy bout of malarial fever, appear fairly continuous. These ... cases have been forwarded to Goroka, and it is hoped that a diagnosis and a course of immediate treatment will be made available here for future reference.[54]

Villagers told him that such people died 'fairly rapidly'. The next year Carey used the term 'kuru' for the sorcery that was killing people, especially the Fore women.[55] The Berndts noticed the sickness, and mentioned it in their first publication of 1952. It was, they said, 'a shaking sickness caused by sorcery'. McArthur in December 1953 and W.T. Brown early in 1954 described the disease accurately.[56] Brown connected 'keru' with sorcery usually by men against women, but sometimes by men against men, and he described how the sorcery 'parcel' was left in a swamp to bring about a 'cold' lingering illness. In May 1955 Colman said that at Magorti

> the wife of the Tul Tul was found in the village sitting dejectedly shaking violently all over (No doubt he [the *tutltul*] will have a vivid picture of the powers of sorcery to carry through his life.). This woman was apparently the victim of 'Kuru'. Later the Tul Tul was interviewed but he had no idea who the sorcerer was. He said he had investigated every bit of swampy ground without success—trying to find the buried personal article taken from his wife.[57]

Colman sent a 'typical' kuru case to Kainantu where the patient was observed by Dr Vincent Zigas. His provisional diagnosis was 'acute hysteria in an otherwise perfectly healthy woman'.[58]

To the government officers kuru, with its direct associations with malign sorcery, accusations and murder, was an impediment to orderly administration rather than a disease. By 1955 victims of kuru had been seen by doctors in Goroka and Kainantu. Gunther says it is likely that by then they knew of kuru in the Department of Public Health in Port Moresby, and Macfarlane Burnet, Director of the Walter and Eliza Hall Institute in Melbourne, said that he heard of the disease in 1955.[59] The disease was a puzzle to those who saw it, but the general explanation was that it was a hysterical condition resulting from a belief in sorcery. The Fore firmly believed it was caused by sorcery.

So kuru was known to Australians for at least six years before it was seen as a health problem, an obligation and an opportunity.

Dr Vincent Zigas, government medical officer at Kainantu, spent twenty days in the Fore in October and November 1956, and on Christmas Day 1956 he wrote his main report to Gunther, the Director of Public Health. Zigas was born in Estonia in 1920, went to school in Helsinki and to universities in Lithuania and Germany.[60] His father, he says, was German and his mother eastern Finnish. He graduated from Hamburg during the war and served as a doctor with the German forces. He was one of the first and youngest of the refugee doctors to arrive in Port Moresby in 1950. By 1956 he was a naturalized Australian. Of his life he says he was not a victim of events beyond his control—he chose where he wanted to go. He was competent, romantic, Quixotic. When he came to write his memories of these times, which he did several times, he shifted between fact, poetic licence and fantasy. He has been called a 'showman' and 'raconteur', and the conscious stylist.[61] For the writer there is always the temptation to quote Zigas because he was involved as worker and observer for so long, and his rambling prose is invested with arresting images, wit and comments of scarifying frankness on his fellows. The historian is inhibited from quoting Zigas because of the uncertain intent of his writings, the uncertain accuracy, and libel laws. When writing of Zigas I have kept to contemporary documents.[62]

Zigas suggested to Gunther in his Christmas letter of 1956 that he be allowed to continue to investigate what he called a 'form of encephalitis'.[63] And he asked that he be allowed to cooperate in research with Dr Anderson to whom he had already sent blood and brain samples.[64] He mentioned Gray Anderson of the Hall Institute because Anderson had recently done important work on Murray Valley Encephalitis in Papua, and while there had helped define the movement of that disease between mosquitoes and birds. In 1955 Gunther had actually been at the Hall Institute talking with Burnet about further research in Papua New Guinea, and both were keen for more work in the Territory. Gunther wrote to Anderson asking him to come up, and indicating that he was ready to make a formal request to the Minister for Territories. In his reply Anderson said he was certainly interested in working on the aetiology of the disease. By February 1957 Burnet and the Hall Board had agreed that Anderson should work on kuru. Anderson set out steps to be followed when samples were sent to him, but had personal and practical reasons delaying his trip north.

The man who did go north was D. Carleton Gajdusek. Born in New York, he was the son of a 'Slovak farm boy' who migrated to America and became a butcher in Yonkers. His mother was the daughter of Hungarian immigrants. From an early age Gajdusek knew that he wanted to be a medical scientist. He was a science prodigy. He graduated in science from Rochester University in 1943, and still only nineteen he entered Harvard Medical School. He did his internship and residency at New York and Cincinnati, specializing in paediatrics. Through the next decade he held a number of posts, from Harvard to California. He also worked for the Department of the Army, and he travelled to Germany, Turkey and Iran and elsewhere. In November 1954 he wrote in a letter that John Enders, Joseph Smadel and Linus Pauling, all his bosses at one time, had won the Nobel Prize. 'Burnet', he wrote, 'will be next'.[65] And he had decided to work with Burnet at the Hall Institute as a visiting fellow.

He took a long time to get there. Burnet had not met Gajdusek before he took up his position at the Hall Institute, and he was puzzled when Gajdusek disappeared for several months. Then he got a cable from Gajdusek in Singapore saying that he could not get a passage on a boat because of the Melbourne Cup. Later Burnet learnt that before getting to Singapore Gajdusek had been wandering the borders of Afghanistan looking for what he called 'opportunistic investigations of epidemiological problems in exotic and isolated populations'.[66] He strayed on to an air base and was retained by the Russians. Gajdusek eventually caught a boat, but got off in Perth and spent several days visiting Aboriginal communities. He arrived in Melbourne on a Saturday and Burnet invited him to his home on the Sunday for a meal. He began talking and talked for hours. At one stage Burnet caught the look of alarm on his wife's face: Gajdusek had been sitting for three-quarters of an hour with an untouched dish in front of him. Gajdusek talked on a wide range of subjects, drew on his prodigious memory, and spoke at a level surpassed only by those who were experts on those subjects. Later, Burnet praised Gajdusek's work at the Hall Institute, interrupted as it was by trips to Cape York, New Britain and Papua where he studied disease patterns, child development, and anything.[67]

In February 1957 Gajdusek left the Hall Institute and he arrived in Port Moresby in early March. He had heard about kuru in Melbourne—for Anderson had been contacted and the first brain and blood samples had arrived before he left—and he talked about kuru in Port Moresby with officials of the Department of Public Health. In Port Moresby the Department of Health believed he was on his way to Lufa. By strange linkages of time and place, Lufa is just to the west of Okapa in the Eastern Highlands, and the government officer then at Lufa was Ian Burnet, the son of Macfarlane. But Gajdusek went straight to Kainantu, met Zigas, saw kuru patients, and Gajdusek and Zigas went to Okapa. Zigas and Gajdusek plunged into research on kuru, and tried to meet other medical demands of the people in the area.

The disease of kuru was more common than previously thought and many of the victims were children. Gajdusek believed that with his knowledge of virology, paediatrics and neurology, he could play a particularly useful role, or roles. His restless mind and restless body drove him to work ceaselessly. He was indifferent to his own physical comfort, walked vast distances, quickly began learning to speak Fore, and filled pages and scraps of paper with his notes.

He said he was preparing the way for Anderson and anxiously awaiting his arrival. He probably was, but within three days of getting to Okapa he was writing of an 'astonishing illness' that would be of interest to the whole medical world. He was going to be at Okapa for months, he said. 'I intend to stick this one out a bit'.[68] On 3 April he assured Joe Smadel he had 'the "real thing" in [his] hands' and he would 'stake his entire medical reputation on this matter'. The exotic wildness and isolation of Okapa meant that for personal and professional reasons there 'could be no better setting in the world for the study of such a disorder'. To leave, he said, would be 'fatal to the project I have fallen into'.[69] He was captured by the place, problem and possibilities. In a letter dated 6 March, but probably 6 April (that is three weeks after arriving at Okapa) he wrote in capitals of the KURU RESEARCH PROJECT at Okapa where work was continuing 'at full speed'.[70]

Gajdusek was sending material to Melbourne for testing, and he was writing to the Public Health Department in Port Moresby for all sorts of medicines, pieces of equipment to be used in post-mortems (such as a knife to cut brains out of skulls), reference books, and buildings, especially a place for autopsies as they were doing them in the bush material room where the patrol officer held court cases.

Here then was a strange situation. Gajdusek had ended his ties with the Hall Institute. He had no position with the Public Health Department in the Territory. He had no funds coming from elsewhere. But he was behaving as if he had standing with both the Hall Institute and the Department, and he was directing a major research project. He had also moved in ahead of Anderson. Roy Scragg, who had taken over from Gunther as Director of Public Health just a few weeks earlier, radioed him suggesting that he withdraw. Gajdusek said no, 'investigation uninterruptable and will remain at work with patients to whom we are responsible'. Burnet wrote a blunt letter to Gajdusek and said Gajdusek's actions were 'indefensible'.[71] Gunther, as Assistant Administrator, followed with a stronger letter in which he accused Gajdusek of claiming to represent the Hall Institute when he did not, and he said that moving into a research project allocated to someone else without prior approval was 'grossly unethical'.[72]

Gajdusek did not seem greatly disturbed by these accusations, and he explained that in fact he had wanted to look at other things in New Guinea, that practical factors had prevented him from going to Lufa. He again said that he was preparing the way for Anderson, that there was enough work for a dozen researchers, and in a few weeks he was unlikely to exhaust all opportunities on a project that would last several years and have universal ramifications. He went on working, but sent more of his material for laboratory analysis to America, and secured institutional backing from America. Typically, Gajdusek had failed to tell the Hall Institute that he was also sending brains to the United States for examination. When Graeme Robertson of the Royal Melbourne Hospital (who was reporting on the brain sections for the Hall Institute) found out that similar work was also being done at the National Institutes of Health in Maryland, he was 'baffled' and thought it 'reprehensible', but accepted his reduced and repetitive role philosophically: 'science must go on'.[73] Anderson did eventually visit Okapa (Gajdusek said he was there for half an hour)[74] and he reported on 16 May 1957.[75] He listed factors that he thought might be significant in the aetiology of kuru: a) genetic factors, b) heavy metal poisoning, and at g) was cannibalism.

Macfarlane Burnet was now inclined to withdraw from kuru research. He was more involved with other issues, and he did not think that a virus was involved (or not the sort of virus that the Hall Institute was accustomed to finding). The Hall Institute continued to carry out tests, but in September Burnet said that that too would end.[76]

In mid-1957 when several scientists were working among the Fore the Acting District Officer for the Eastern Highlands, W. (Bill) Tomasetti, wrote to the Director, Department of Native Affairs, that kuru was 'almost certainly not one of the major Territory health problems'.⁷⁷ The caution of the *kiaps* was in contrast to the enthusiastic possessiveness of the scientists. Given the different perspectives, responsibilities and opportunities of *kiaps* and scientists both were right.

Gajdusek was now the dominant researcher, and his lines of practical and intellectual support were American. The Administrator, Donald Cleland, wrote that he regretted that Gajdusek was shifting so much material to America, that clearly the next stage of the work would be done in the United States, and that much of the research done by Gajdusek in the Territory could have been carried out by a 'qualified Australian worker'.⁷⁸ Gunther and Burnet were less confident that someone else would have done as much and as well. Gunther said of the man whom he accused of usurping a research project, 'Thank God he did'.

In November 1957 Gajdusek and Zigas published the first scholarly articles defining kuru. The article in the *New England Journal of Medicine* came out before the one in the *Medical Journal of Australia*. That priority of publishing, too, annoyed some Australians, and it was true that Gajdusek was determined to publish first in America.⁷⁹

The progress of the disease was now clear. The sufferers were themselves the first to know that they had kuru: they lost balance and had to support themselves by clutching neighbours or using a stick. They developed a tremor that intensified, and they suffered some tendon jerks, involuntary laughter, and blurred speech. Eventually they lost the ability to walk, even to sit up, and finally they became incontinent and unable to swallow. The whole process took a few months, rarely a year. That was fast for a degenerative disease. All cases were fatal.[80] Those most likely to suffer the disease were children of both sexes and adult women. The youngest child with the disease was about four. In postmortems, the brains of kuru victims were found to suffer widespread degeneration, especially in the cerebellum.

This fragment of the kuru narrative has concentrated on the question of who owned the research. That whole dispute was repeated in 1959 with more vitriol when Gajdusek was in conflict with J.H. Bennett, Professor of Genetics from Adelaide University, and what was generally known as the Adelaide group.[81]

Simultaneously, another public health issue with its own moral implications became critical. It was the decision to fence the Fore.

Bennett and his co-authors suggested in 1958 that there was a possible genetic basis for kuru, and in October 1959 after analysis of two hundred pedigrees Bennett made a much stronger case that kuru was determined by genes.[82] He said that the existence of particular genes explained the pattern of incidence. In December he wrote a letter pointing out that the movement of men out of the kuru region meant that in twenty or so years there would be a serious health problem right across the highlands, and indeed in the whole of New Guinea.[83] In spite of his warnings, he said, nothing had been done to make a record of all those Fore who had left the region, and more Fore were leaving. With the imbalance in men to women in the Fore this exodus was likely to quicken.

A committee chaired by Burnet reviewed Bennett's work and decided that while kuru was 'essentially genetic' they thought it was impractical and a denial of rights to quarantine the Fore.

The recommendations of the committee went to John Gunther. He was faced with strong advice from Bennett, a leading Australian geneticist, and the statistical evidence was alarming. In between the censuses of August 1958 and January 1960, that is, in less than eighteen months, the population of the South Fore had dropped by two point four percent. In the adult population males outnumbered females by two thousand five hundred and sixty-two to one thousand one hundred and sixty-three. Gunther thought that kuru might be killing half the females and one in ten of the males. Kuru, he wrote, was such a 'foul disease', Australian officials were obliged to try to contain it. And they would.[84]

He therefore went back to the Burnet committee, contacted each member separately, and got them to agree that they should try to fence the Fore. They would let no one out, and they would return all those who had left. That was five hundred and twenty-nine Fore and perhaps one thousand in total from the whole affected area had to be sent home. They were all over the place, including serving in the Pacific Islands Regiment. They would be returned to a situation where, because there were two men for every woman, most could never marry, and where prospects for an education or chances to earn cash were slight. There would therefore have to be compensating economic and social policies implemented immediately in the Fore.

The Minister for Territories, Paul Hasluck, accepted the proposals. For the first time the government would attempt to quarantine a gene. The legislation was drafted—but nothing happened.

While the administrative steps were being taken, Gunther searched the world for reassessments of Bennett's gene explanation. The experts told him they could not accept Bennett's findings on his published material: they would need to review his data. But several expressed doubts, and those doubts gradually became stronger. The genetic theory did not explain why some of those with the gene did not manifest the disease (the failure of penetrance), the death rate was so high that the gene should have been eliminating itself, there was not sufficient consistency in siblings and in other close blood relationships, there was difficulty explaining the frequency of deaths in both male and female children and only in adult females, and there seemed to be cases of Fore men marrying women from outside the kuru region, bringing them back, and then they contracted kuru.[85] The notion that some people had a genetic disposition continued, but a gene as primary cause faded.[86] The Fore just escaped the fence.

Another complex moral issue deserving examination is the rights of the Fore when their living and dead were being subjected to many tests, and when Fore sick, dead and parts of bodies were being taken from home hamlets. Scientists and administrators also had rights and responsibilities, certainly to secure the health and welfare of the Fore and of peoples beyond Okapa. The unfettered (or fettered) right to pursue knowledge is less clear. The question of the rights and interests of the sick, the officials and the scientists on a frontier of knowledge, culture contact, administrative control and nationality has been set aside here. After the research has been done and the results published there remains the question of who is given the credit, even which discipline is credited.

Bob Glasse was an American anthropologist who did his doctorate at the Australian National University—he was one of the first of the anthropologists into the highlands.[87] Shirley Inglis went to Melbourne University then did a diploma in anthropology at Sydney. Soon after Bob and Shirley were married they went to do fieldwork in the Fore, initially supported by the Genetics Department of the University of Adelaide.[88] In 1961 they set up house at Wanitabe where they worked on kinship, the origin and spread of kuru, sorcery, what they thought relevant, and the topics the Fore opened to them as they sat about the Glasses' house.

One day Bob was reading the *Time* magazine of 18 May 1962. In it there was a report that if you trained a flatworm to respond to an electric flash, then chopped it up and fed the pieces to another flatworm, the cannibal flatworm acquired the memory of the trained flatworm. Bob asked, how would that be for a model for kuru? And, Shirley remembers, 'we laughed ourselves silly'.[89] But over the next few days various strands of knowledge began to weave into one.[90] They knew that kuru was a recent disease. In fact it was possible to map village to village the appearance of the first case, starting about 1921 and going through to the 1940s. Cannibalism had also been adopted recently, and there was a correlation with kuru following cannibalism.[91] The Fore ate their own dead: they rarely ate enemy dead. Men thought that to eat human flesh was dangerous and that it weakened them. And men could afford to reject some protein because they ate most of the pork.[92] But as the forests and the hunting declined, the Fore women were short of protein. Children lived and ate with their mothers, but when boys at seven shifted to the men's house they ate with the men. Fore cannibalism was not ritual cannibalism, it did not have the clear rules, the ceremony or the symbolic significance of ritual, but some parts of the corpse were normally eaten by certain female relatives. The brain and almost all of the body were consumed.

In their study of Fore genealogies the Glasses had also shown that the Fore were not dominated by relationships determined by birth: relationships could be made and children were adopted.

So here was an explanation that appeared to fit the observed phenomena: kuru was a disease of children and adult women, and it appeared to be, but was not quite, hereditary. Obviously if cannibalism was the means of transmission then the sons and daughters of women who contracted the disease were likely to get the disease. They all ate together, and the adopted children were as vulnerable as those who were of direct descent. And here, too, was an explanation why the youngest children were no longer getting kuru. In the North Fore no children born since about 1951 had kuru, and cannibalism had been suppressed longer in the north.

Macfarlane Burnet heard the explanation in a thatched roof hut at Wanitabe and was sceptical. It was too 'pretty', too precise, and answers were rarely that tidy. And, he said, there was a million to one chance involved: the agent had to appear in the Fore right at that time that they were adopting cannibalism. Other people to their north who were cannibals and had been cannibals for hundreds and hundreds of years did not suffer from kuru.

Cannibalism fitted with another factor. In 1959 W.J. Hadlow had published a letter in *The Lancet* pointing out that kuru was similar to scrapie in sheep, and scrapie was transmissible by inoculation. In 1963 Gajdusek inoculated chimpanzees with material from the brains of kuru sufferers and in 1966 the first chimpanzee manifested kuru. Some agent of kuru, then called a slow or latent virus, was being transmitted.

The Glasses produced typed papers setting out the significance of cannibalism, but they did not publish their findings for some years. In fact they did not make their first comprehensive published statement for five years.[93] That is one reason why their imaginative link of kuru and cannibalism is often given slight attention or completely omitted.[94] Different behaviour in different disciplines may also be a factor. Anthropologists own their research, even possess the people they research, and many of their findings are specific to those people. They are often quick to talk and slow to publish, and competition to be first to publish is not strong when all are dealing with different subjects.

Much research and many issues have been omitted in this brief survey. The first narrative directs attention to the question of who owns a research project and the significance of nationalism and personality in deciding possession. Several of the main characters involved were sharply distinctive and the conflict between nations was being decided on or beyond the Australian frontier where the Australians wanted monuments to their presence. Through those four years of dispute Vin Zigas was in an invidious position. He wanted to do good but was pulled in different directions by his commitment to the Department of Public Health that had given him his chance to practise medicine and which he continued to serve, by his friendship and admiration for Carleton Gajdusek, and by his commitment to his new nation of Australia—which had only partly accepted him.

In the second narrative there is the question of the responsibility of health administrators when they thought they had a lethal gene to control. It is also interesting that the widely accepted genetic explanation lost favour before any particular scholar wrote a sustained rejection.[95]

The third raises questions about the process by which explanations are made, and speculates on vagaries of attribution.

Think again of the Fore and their near neighbours who had suffered two thousand and five hundred deaths from kuru by 1977. In 1957 they had faced not just revolution but extinction. They exhorted one another to give up the sorcery that was killing them. They made sad pilgrimages to charlatans among them and their neighbours who claimed to have a cure.[96] Men whose first and then second wives had died struggled to garden, feed children and tend pigs. The whole structure of the society was under stress. And for all the intensity, rivalry, imagination and chauvinism that went into the research, for all the success of the research, no kuru sufferer was saved.

In May 1951 the acting Assistant District Officer at Kainantu, G. Linsley, had written about the Fore eating their own dead, and that near Moke (Okapa) the people said they no longer did so because the missionaries had told them it was wrong. Further south, Linsley said, the people made no attempt to conceal their cannibalism: they freely discussed how bodies were consumed and that even the bones were pounded so that they too could be eaten.[97] Linsley doubted that the people near Okapa had so quickly given up cannibalism: he suspected that they knew that the white men disapproved of the practice and so unlike their less knowing neighbours to the south they would no longer talk about it. In 1951 on the west of the Fore in the Wamu valley, Carey and McArthur reported:

> Cannibalism is very rampant in the area. It is the custom of these people to eat their dead. Burial grounds are not in existence. The police on the stations in the area have done their utmost to prevent the custom, but to no avail. We instructed all the luluais who were provisionally appointed that they must set aside an area suitable for a burial ground, and that when a person died, he was to be buried in this marked area. [T]he person could not, under any circumstances be eaten. This information at the first [sic] seemed not to their liking; but they finally promised to do as we had told them. Police were instructed to take the next offenders into custody, and escort them into GOROKA.[98]

The next year Desailly investigated a case where two women were said to have dug up a freshly buried corpse of a dead child, and were about to prepare it for consumption. Desailly decided that there was insufficient evidence to charge the women, and in any case taking the two women away for trial or punishment would have caused trouble. He 'addressed' the people 'on the subject of eating the dead', and they agreed that it was wrong, and that in the past they had sometimes buried bodies according to instructions, but later dug them up.[99]

McArthur, back in the Wamu valley in 1952, found from checking the census, that a man had died. The people told him that the man had been buried, but later McArthur learnt this was untrue. The bones of the man were lying on a stick bed in a tree. While in the past the people had sometimes left bodies in trees to decompose, McArthur decided that in this case the bones were not in a natural position, and on the ground under the body were none of the worms that usually flourished on the bits of decaying corpse falling through the platform. McArthur thought that the body had probably been eaten, but nobody was prepared to say so. Cannibalism had declined in frequency, McArthur said, but continued hidden from the government. He thought it might be worthwhile for later patrols to check some graves to make sure that they did indeed contain bodies.[100]

In fact, the Fore were rapidly abandoning cannibalism. Under persuasion, threat and choice, other groups too were giving up the practice, although some Gimi on the west of the Fore persisted for a few years after the first census patrols. The Native Regulation that people were to bury their dead in an appropriate place outside the village was one of the first and most universally imposed government rules.[101] It was the incidental effect of this 'Reg', and *kiap* and mission teaching, that would eventually end the pestilence. Forty years after Zigas and Gajdusek described kuru for the medical world, the incidence of the disease has fallen to two or three cases a year, and all those recent victims were infants at cannibal meals close to the time of contact.[102]

A final word on Gajdusek. At the height of the second controversy when some people wanted him excluded from the research area, Ian Holmes Acting District Officer, Eastern Highlands wrote:

> Though loquacious, authoritative and categorical [Gajdusek] strikes the impartial observer as an extremely active and enthusiastic man who puts up with considerable hardship in the interests of research.

He is popular with natives and displays keen interest in their customs, attitudes, welfare and administration. He actively co-operates with the Administration in the field, although is sometimes outspoken in *his* opinions regarding the uninhibited rights of legitimate research workers.[103]

In 1976 Gajdusek and Baruch Blumberg were jointly awarded the Nobel prize in physiology and medicine. It was for 'discoveries concerning new mechanisms for the origin and dissemination of infectious diseases'.

In 1957 when Carleton Gajdusek went to Okapa he was thirty-three, he knew he had more energy, more imagination and a greater breadth of learning than most of his fellow researchers. He wanted to do something great, he wanted recognition for that achievement, and—after a time—he passionately wanted to do good for the Fore. Kuru was his opportunity and he seized it. Strangely that restless, wide-ranging mind did not make the early unorthodox connections—with scrapie and with cannibalism.[104] But he deserved his prize. He played a central role in showing that an agent was being transmitted (at first called a slow, latent or unorthodox virus) and that kuru was related to other degenerative diseases of the central nervous system, perhaps to Alzheimer's disease. The presumption now is that the infective agent is a prion, and it causes the protein in the brain to replicate in aberrant form, reducing the brain to vacuoles (spongiform) and plaques. The presumed transmission in the hysteria over Mad Cow Disease was from scrapie infected sheep converted into a concentrated food for cattle. Scrapie manifested itself in the cattle as BSE, and when humans ate the the beef of infected cattle they contracted CJD, an illness similar to kuru. That chain of presumption about 'prion' diseases goes back to hamlets of the Fore and their encounter with the brilliance, opportunism, selfishness, service and self-effacement of western science.

ACKNOWLEDGEMENTS

I am grateful to Ken Inglis for his comments on a draft of this paper.

NOTES

[1] Parts of this article were first presented as a talk at the National Academies Forum and Humanities Research Centre seminar, Mad Cows and Modernity, Australian National University, 25 May 1996, and it was then prepared for publication in the *Journal of Pacific History*, Vol 32 No 2, 1996, pp.178-201.

[2] The most comprehensive reports have been in the Washington Post, 26 and 27 April 1996.

[3] The combined territories were known in 1957 as the Territory of Papua and New Guinea. The 'and' between Papua and New Guinea was omitted in 1971 and the independent nation created in 1975 became 'Papua New Guinea'. I have sometimes called the people of the Territory 'Papua New Guineans'. It is anachronistic, but convenient, to use that term before 1971.

[4] Annual Reports have figures and maps.

[5] It is surprising how few police went on many long patrols. Skinner in 1947 had fifteen (5 of 1947/8, Kainantu), but Timperley in 1948 had just six (4 of 1948/9, Kainantu), and McArthur on a very long patrol, 19 May-8 July 1952, had just five police (10 of 1952/3, Goroka). Skinner was entering much new country, but Timperley and McArthur were in areas where the people had only brief encounters with the outside world.

[6] Annual Report 1956-7, p.20.

[7] Figures in Annual Reports, and they are set out in Ian Downs, The Australian Trusteeship: Papua New Guinea 1945-75, Australian Government Publishing Service, Canberra, 1980, p.122.

[8] J.Lee, 'The New Guinea Elite', <u>The Journal of the Papua & New Guinea Society</u>, Vol 1 No 2, 1967, pp.113-7.

[9] Gunther in recorded interviews with H.Nelson beginning on 2 November 1971, and a typescript, Post-war Medical Services in Papua New Guinea—a personal view, held by H.Nelson.

[10] <u>Annual Report</u>, for Papua, 1956-7, p.23.

[11] <u>Annual Reports</u>, 1956-7, New Guinea 1422 patients (p.89), and Papua 641 (pp.71 and 72).

[12] The Minister for Territories, Paul Hasluck argued that the relationship was unique.

[13] It was spelt 'Forei' By R.I.Skinner in 1947, but it was usually 'Fore' by the time G.Toogood was there in August 1949.

[14] There are several summaries of the Fore: D.C.Gajdusek and M.Alpers, 'Genetic Studies in Relation to Kuru. I. Cultural, Historical, and Demographic Background', <u>The American Journal of Human Genetics</u>, Vol 24 No 6, part II, November 1972, pp.S1-S38; R.W.Hornabrook, ed., <u>Essays on Kuru</u>, Classey, Faringdon, 1976 (several chapters); and S.Lindenbaum, <u>Kuru Sorcery: Disease and danger in the New Guinea Highlands</u>, Mayfield, Palo Alto, 1979.

[15] V.Zigas, <u>Laughing Death: The untold story of Kuru</u>, Humana Press, Clifton, New Jersey, 1990, p.143.

[16] R.Radford, <u>Highlanders and Foreigners in the Upper Ramu: The Kainantu area 1919-1942</u>, Melbourne University Press, Melbourne, 1987, outlines the movements of government officers, prospectors and miners in the area.

[17] Cadet Patrol Officer K.I.Morgan inspected a crashed American plane near Moke in 1951, and he wondered whether the five bombs still there were dangerous. Kainantu Patrol Report, 7 of 1950/51.

[18] D.S.Grove, Kainantu Patrol Report, 3 of 1947/48.

[19] There were cases of Papua New Guinean police and soldiers being persuaded, or feeling obliged, to use their rifles in surreptitious support of particular communities in tribal disputes.

[20] R.I.Skinner, Kainantu Patrol Report, 5 of 1947/48.

[21] R.I.Skinner, Kainantu Patrol Report, 5 of 1947/48.

22 K.J.Morgan, Kainantu Patrol Report, 7 of 1950/51.

23 G.Linsley, Kainantu Patrol Report, 8 of 1950/51.

24 Goroka Patrol Report, 4 of 1950/51.

25 R.N.Desailly, Goroka Patrol Report, 10 of 1951/52.

26 G.W.Toogood, Kainantu Patrol Report, 5 of 1949/50.

27 H.W.West, Kainantu Patrol Report, 5 of 1953/54.

28 John McArthur had a motor bike.

29 G.Toogood and K.J.Morgan, Kainantu Patrol Reports, 2 of 1950/51.

30 W.J.Kelly, Kainantu Patrol Report, 8 of 1951/52.

31 W.J. Kelly, Kainantu Patrol Report, 8 of 1951/52. John Colman opposed the change from traditional dress to the laplap. He said he was having a 'drive' against the change, and was pleased when people reported for the census in traditional dress. (Kainantu Patrol Report, 6 of 1955/56) But the Fore were also influenced by the 'traditional dress of those further north and longer contacted.

32 H.W.West, Kainantu Patrol Report, 5 of 1953/4.

33 W.J.Kelly, Kainantu Patrol Report, 8 of 1951/52.

34 John McArthur, Kainantu Patrol Report, 4 of 1954/55.

35 Jack Baker, Kainantu Patrol Report, 6 of 1956/7. In 1955 John McArthur noted that four villages had coffee plots, about 500 trees in all, and he issued them with crotalaria (shade tree) seeds. (4 of 1954/55).

36 Herwig Wagner and Hermann Reiner, eds, <u>The Lutheran Church in Papua New Guinea</u>, Lutheran Publishing House, Adelaide, 1986, p.228. Albert and Sylvia Frerichs, <u>Anutu Conquers in New Guinea: A story of mission work in New Guinea</u>, Augsburg Publishing House, Minnesota, 1969. Early missionaries in charge of Tarabo station were Diemer, Fiegert and Bamler. E.A.Jericho, <u>Seedtime and Harvest in New Guinea</u>, New Guinea Mission Board, 1961(?).

37 Jack Baker, Kainantu Patrol Report, 6 of 1956/57.

38 W.J.Kelly, Kainantu Patrol Report, 8 of 1951/52.

39 H.W.West, Kainantu Patrol Report, 5 of 1953/54.

40 W.J.Kelly, Kainantu Patrol Report, 8 of 1951/52.

41 H.W.West, Kainantu Patrol Report, 8 of 1952/53.

42 H.W.West, Kainantu Patrol Report, 5 of 1953/54.

43 G.Linsley, Kainantu Patrol Report, 8 of 1950/51. John Colman said that if a New Guinean around Kainantu disappeared for a few days the rumour was that he had gone to the Fore to get information about sorcery or to hire a sorcerer. (Kainantu Patrol Report, 14 of 1954/55).

44 G.Linsley, Kainantu Patrol Report, 8 of 1950/51. Wood was being replaced by wire. The <u>Tok Pisin</u> term, <u>sutim nil</u>, (injecting nails) was used.

45 W.J.Kelly, Kainantu Patrol Report, 8 of 1951/52.

46 John McArthur, Kainantu Patrol Report, 4 of 1954/55.

47 John Colman, Kainantu Patrol Report, 14 of 1954/55.

48 John McArthur, Kainantu Patrol Report, 4 of 1954/55.

49 Glasse and Lindenbaum, 'Kuru at Wanitabe', in R.W.Hornabrook, ed., <u>Essays on Kuru</u>, Classey, Faringdon, 1976, p.46.

50 R.M.Berndt, 'A cargo movement in the Eastern Highlands of New Guinea', <u>Oceania</u>, 1952-53, Vol 23 No 1, pp.40-65, No 2 pp.137-158, and No 3 pp.202-234; <u>Oceania</u>, 'Reaction to Contact in the Eastern Highlands of New Guinea', 1953-54, Vol 24 No 3, pp.190-228 and No 4, pp.255-274; <u>Excess and Restraint</u>, University of Chicago Press, Chicago, 1962.

51 H.W.West, Kainantu Patrol Report, 5 of 1953/54. By the time the second census was taken the fact that men greatly outnumbered women in many villages was obvious. Government officers did not draw attention to this, presumably because they thought that women were over-represented among those who chose not to be censused.

52 There was also an airstrip at Tarabo.

53 J.D.Mathews, Kuru: A puzzle in cultural and environmental medicine, Doctor of Medicine thesis, University of Melbourne, 1971, has a survey of early contact.

54 Arthur Carey, Goroka Patrol Report, 4 of 1950/51. Kauna, in the Yate language group, is within the northern edge of the kuru area. The temperature is oddly low, but kuru was afebrile. Earlier Carey said that he was told the condition started with 'stomach trouble'. That was not a symptom of kuru.

55 Mathews, Kuru, p.11.

56 W.T.Brown, Kainantu Patrol Report, 8 of 1953/54. Brown, who patrolled in January and February 1954, wrote: 'The first sign of impending death is a general debility which is followed by general weakness and inability to stand. The victim retires to her house. She is able to take a little nourishment but suffers from violent shivering. The next stage is that the victim lies down in the house and cannot take nourishment and death eventually ensures[sic].' Brown used the term 'keru', and described fairly accurately 'keru' sorcery and divination. (Appendix B to Patrol Report). J.D.Mathews, Kuru 1971, pp.11-2, refers to A.T.Carey's patrol of 1951 and to McArthur's of 1953.

57 John Colman, Kainantu Patrol Report, 14 of 1954/55.

58 H.W.West to District Commissioner, Eastern Highlands, 8 July 1955, with Colman's report, 14 of 1954/55.

59 Macfarlane Burnet in recorded interview with H.Nelson, 25 January 1977.

60 Zigas wrote two books, Auscultation of Two Worlds, Vantage Press, New York, 1978; and Laughing Death: The untold story of Kuru, Humana Press, Clifton, New Jersey, 1990. He also wrote survey articles such as 'Kuru: A critical review', Medical Journal of Australia, 2, 20 September 1975. Carleton Gajdusek wrote an obituary of him in Neurology, 33 September 1983, pp.1199-1200.

61 The quoted words are from Gajdusek's foreword to Vincent Zigas, Laughing Death. In the Foreword Gajdusek wrestles with defining Zigas's works of reminiscence and imagination.

62 In his article 'Kuru: A Critical Review' in the Medical Journal of Australia, 20 September 1975, p.483, Zigas says he went to the Fore area early in 1955, found nine cases, made an official report early in 1956, was granted permission to spend more time in the Fore etc. Some of this may be true, but all is inconsistent with the facts that Colman sent two cases of kuru to Zigas in mid 1955, that Zigas then diagnosed them as suffering from hysteria, that his report of 25 December 1956 describing his recent patrol into the Fore indicates that this was his first encounter with kuru in the Fore area, and that in the December report he requested permission to investigate the disease.

[63] Generally Gunther was not a diary writer or a keeper of copies of government files, but among his papers he did preserve three files on kuru research and development in the Okapa area. Those three files are now held by H.Nelson.

[64] Macfarlane Burnet, Walter and Eliza Hall Institute 1915-1965, Melbourne University Press, Melbourne, 1971, pp.136-8.

[65] Carleton Gajdusek, A Year in the Middle East: Expeditions in Iran and Afghanistan with travels in Europe and North Africa 1954, National Institutes of Health, Bethesda, 1991, p.389. Through the National Institutes Health Gajdusek published some 5000 densely written pages of his journals—often on expeditions relating to his kuru research. In addition he released Correspondence on the Discovery and Original Investigations on Kuru: Smadel-Gajdusek correspondence 1955-1958, National Institutes of Health, Bethesda, 1976; and Judith Farquhar and D.C.Gajdusek, eds, Kuru: Early letters and field-notes from the collection of D.Carleton Gajdusek, Raven Press, New York, 1981. Probably no scientist has been so open, so prolific and so articulate. Burnet was not the next to win the Nobel, but he got it in 1960.

[66] Gajdusek in preface to 'Unconventional Viruses and the Origin and Disappearance of Kuru', Nobel Lecture, NIH, Maryland, 1976, p.165.

[67] MacfarlaneBurnet, Walter and Eliza Hall Institute 1915-1965, Melbourne University Press, Melbourne, 1971, p.144; and recorded interview.

[68] Gajdusek to Smadel, 15 March 1957, Correspondence, pp.50-1.

[69] Gajdusek to Smadel, 3 April 1957, Correspondence, pp.66-7.

[70] Gajdusek to Scragg, 6 March 1957, Kuru file, Gunther papers.

[71] Burnet to Gajdusek, 26 March 1957, Kuru file, Gunther Papers.

[72] Gunther to Gajdusek, 9 April 1957, Kuru file, Gunther Papers.

[73] Robertson to J.G.Greenfield, 31 October 1957, Correspondence, p.305.

[74] Gajdusek to Smadel, no date, Correspondence, p.88.

[75] Gunther Papers, Kuru file.

[76] Burnet to Scragg, 25 September 1957, Kuru file, Gunther Papers. Some work continued in Australia eg by the CSIRO and at the Baker Institute.

77 W. Tomasetti to Director, Dept of Native Affairs, 31 July 1957, with Kainantu Patrol Report, 6 of 1956/7.

78 Cleland to Secretary, Dept of Territories, no date, but after 25 September 1957, Kuru file, Gunther Papers.

79 An editorial in the Medical Journal of Australia, said, 'Some regret may be felt that work which originated and was developing in Australian hands should be diverted overseas, when it could have been done at least as effectively by Australian investigators'. (23 November 1957, p.765) Gajdusek in fact sent the first draft article to Science, the Journal of the American Association for the Advancement of Science, but the editor there thought it more suited to a medical journal. Smadel sent it to the New England Journal of Medicine. Gajdusek said he submitted the second article to Australia 'for political reasons', but he was 'counting on' the American article being first, and he was ready to 'urge' and 'beg' for that to happen. (Correspondence, pp.145,7,9).

80 This was not then certain. Cases of recovery or remission were often being reported—but not confirmed.

81 I have failed to mention many other early researchers: Charles Julius an anthropologist, Lucy Hamiliton, dietician, Bill Symes, doctor and linguist, A.V.G. Price, pathologist, and others—most sent by or with the assistance of the Department of Public Health.

82 J.H. Bennett, F.A. Rhodes and H.N. Robson, 'Observations on Kuru: I. a possible genetic basis', Australasian Annals of Medicine, Vol 7 No 4, November 1958, pp.269-75; and J.H. Bennett, A.J. Gray and C.O. Auricht, 'The Genetical Study of Kuru', Medical Journal of Australia, 10 October 1959, pp.505-8.

83 Bennett to the Committee of Enquiry into the Handling of the Kuru problem in New Guinea, 15 Dec 1959, Research at Okapa file, Gunther papers. Bennett raised the question of kuru being spread in letters of 15 January to Cleland, and 3 September 1959 to the Administrator. He followed up with a very strong warning to the Administrator on 24 February 1960, Kuru file, Gunther Papers.

84 Report on Kuru and Recommendations for Its Further Investigation and Control, By Gunther, undated but around May 1960, summarized the steps and his responses. Research at Okapa file, Gunther Papers.

85 This indicated that the significant factor was in the Okapa region—either in the physical or social environment. But some Fore developed the disease after they had been away from home for many years. This seemed to preclude a local cause or trigger.

86 Macfarlane Burnet, 'Kuru-The Present Position', <u>Papua and New Guinea Medical Journal</u>, Vol 8, No 1, 1 March 1965, p.4 said that 'Bennett's hypothesis is consistent with all the available data and can be accepted as basically correct', but that there was also another factor acting on the 'genetically susceptible'. He also warned that it was important to monitor the health of the children of Fore men who left the area and married women from elsewhere.

87 Robert Glasse, <u>Huli of Papua: A cognatic descent system</u>, Mouton, Paris and The Hague, 1968.

88 Shirley Inglis became Shirley Glasse then Shirley Lindenbaum.

89 S.Lindenbaum in recorded interview with H.Nelson, 5 September 1978.

90 South Fore Cannibalism and Kuru, a typed paper, was written early in 1962, and presents much of the basic argument. It was the basis for a presentation of their findings in Adelaide in 1962.

91 The Glasses had investigated the history of kuru by the time they made the connection with cannibalism, but much of the history of cannibalism was researched later. Some other evidence was also pursued after it was assumed that cannibalism was a means of transmission. Not all evidence was immediately available to be fitted together.

92 As Shirley Lindenbaum has pointed out there were many exceptions: some strong, aggressive men ignored the fears of other men and took part in cannibal feasts, and not all bodies of relatives were eaten, <u>Kuru Sorcery: Disease and danger in the New Guinea Highlands</u>, Mayfield, Palo Alto, 1979, pp.19-25.

93 Robert Glasse, New York Academy of Sciences, <u>Transactions,</u> Series II, Vol 29 No 6, 1967, pp.748-54; J.D.Mathews, Robert Glasse and Shirley Lindenbaum, 'Kuru and Cannibalism', <u>The Lancet</u>, 24 August 1968, pp.449-52; R.Glasse and S.Lindenbaum, 'Kuru at Wanitabe', in Hornabrook 1976, pp.38-52; and S.Lindenbaum, <u>Kuru Sorcery: Disease and danger in the New Guinea Highlands</u>, Mayfield, Palo Alto, 1979.

94 Burnet in his 1965 paper on 'Kuru-the present position' p.4 said that at a conference in London in 1964 the 'hypothesis that cannibalism may have been involved was only briefly discussed, the general position being that, if it was in any sense relevant, it could only be as an (unlikely) means of disseminating a viral agent.'

95 Norma McArthur, 'The age incidence of kuru', <u>Annals of Human Genetics</u>, 27, 1964, p.352 said that the hypothesis put forward by Bennett et al. in 1959 was 'untenable'. McArthur had gone to New Guinea in 1963 at the request of the Medical Research Advisory Committee.

96 Lindenbaum, <u>Kuru Sorcery</u>, pp.69-72, 100-16.

97 G.Linsley, Kainantu Patrol Report, 8 of 1950/51. The Glasses later made the same point about bones being pounded for consumption.

98 Goroka Patol Report, 1 of 1951/52. The Gimi people of the Wamu valley did not suffer kuru as those to the east did.

99 R.N.Desailly, Goroka Patrol Report, 10 of 1951/52.

100 John McArthur, Goroka Patrol Report, 1 of 1952/53.

101 They were the 'Native Administration Regulations' in New Guinea. The Papuan Regulation dated back to 1890 in British New Guinea.

102 Colin Masters gave current rates of infection at the ANU seminar, Mad Cows and Modernity, on 25 May 1996.

103 Undated, but read by Cleland on 26 August. The year is not written but by the numbering on the file is 1959. Research at Okapa file, Gunther papers.

104 He got close to both. He read veterinary literature on his way home from Okapa, and he was interested in staggers in sheep—but this was a disease induced by <u>Phalaris Tuberosa</u>, it was not scrapie. He often collected information on cannibalism, and in November 1957 he wondered if eating brains might trigger the disease—but rejected the idea as he thought the Fore did not eat brains and that the youngest sufferers had not been involved in the eating of corpses. He was wrong on both points. (<u>Correspondence</u> p.392, pp.300,311)

MAD COW DISEASE:
A BOVINE VIEWPOINT
Robin Wallace-Crabbe

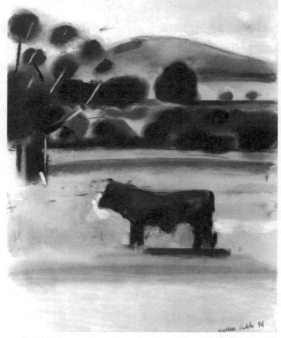

Robin Wallace-Crabbe, *Shorthorn in a Paddock*, 1996

What you notice—at least I noticed, running cattle, rearing calves, being involved with the range of activities which are, I suppose, 'husbandry', assisting when the vet is treating with antibiotics the pizzle of a bull who has torn it on a barb wire fence—what you notice is that cattle display marked individual differences. Their temperaments vary greatly, as does their capacity to establish enduring relationships with other animals within the herd. Kept in isolation from their own kind they may establish a relationship with an animal of another species, though rarely I understand with a tiger. With the onset of disease I have come to believe that a particular animal's character determines its ability to fight the disease. Some take the optimistic view, others just lie down and die. Cows I have nursed, that have suffered damage to a nerve along their spine as a result of a difficult calving, will usually survive if you can get them into a shed and roll them over a couple of times a day until the nerve damage is repaired. But you need to keep up their interest in life at the same time as maintaining their food intake and keeping them warm. So, in those circumstances, several times a day ... blah, blah, blah.

When I was a teenager in Melbourne, we pubescent through to nubile schoolchildren, changing trains or trams in the city, congregated at the Collins Street Swanston Street corner where the Athenaeum Club and the Athenaeum Theatre and the Town Hall and the Regent and the Plaza cinemas and nice shops selling nice things, several selling sweet things, a tobacconist selling pipes and tobacco and Cuban cigars reputed to have been rolled on the thighs of Cuban women of legendary beauty, all existed cheek by jowl, one with the other in such harmony as only exists in lost golden ages. Yes, for real teen style it was Hilliers on Collins Street where a milk shake with nutmeg sprinkled on top was amazing, or a spider was nice, or, if memory proves correct, a waffle with maple syrup cost more money but was alright too. Frappé was for the most sophisticated. To buy a brandy snap meant strolling down what I believe was called Regent Place, a narrow streetlet leading to the hard backside of Saint Paul's Anglican Cathedral. Maybe that narrow streetlet (did it have Tim the Toyman in it?) continued all the way through to Flinders Street, providing a breathing space between the Gas and Fuel Corporation and the fabric of the Cathedral itself. Or was that part called Cathedral Place?

Mating rituals, for the boys and girls changing trains or trams and hanging about the vicinity of Swanston and Collins, were doomed for quite some time yet to lead nowhere. Everybody then had become convinced by various smooth-talking moral authorities that the actual coupling aspect of mating was much too frightening to contemplate, that outside of marriage copulation led to social disenfranchisement and, far worse, we knew too well that adultery led to the fragmentation of wealth—not that we were up to adultery, not yet, we were mere novices at the gateway of the sexual maze. As well there were sexual diseases—bacterial (cocci, spirilla), fungal, parasitic and legendary wee creatures called crabs.

Yet there were pre-mating rituals in which we were all too eager to participate. At Hilliers these involved the ingestion of cow's milk, served up in various bizarre forms, some I have already mentioned. But the greatest form of all, a monument to our human capacity for invention, was the ice-cream sundae. Ah yes, there was with the eating of ice-cream sundaes the having-our-way-with melting icy cow's-milk pleasure domes topped with sweet syrup, chocolate, strawberry, pineapple, banana, caramel, whatever, and sprinkled o'er with nuts. I seem to remember that yellower-than-ice-cream, whipped close to becoming butter was squeezed around the edges of the shallow fluted glass ice-cream sundae serving dish for the extra fat, not to mention decorative effect.

Hilliers was the ultimate mammalian mother, an enormous sow/ bitch/cow reclining on its side with us, the children suckling eagerly upon its milk-weeping teats.

Stage one boy-girl mating rituals for us, then, were sharing a spoon while our faces hovered above the confection, sucking sweet flavoured milk through a straw cheek to cheek, licking sweetened cream from one or other end of a butter rich and brittle brandy snap. Few of us knew better.

Anyway, mating rituals were one thing, but so frightening were the rumoured consequences of a fully executed sexual coupling, and so hideous, dark and forbidden the sweets of our sexuality, that we, the dairy product and sugar addicted young (there was legislation in place supporting both these industries, guaranteeing that we would grow up sugar and milk fixated) who were so sexually excited by the mere touch of an ink stained finger, or observation of a beloved cheek flushed scarlet by unjustified shame and the activities of a sympathetic nervous system driven crazy in a tram within which bodies were so crushed together that had the boys and girls been cattle or sheep, relevant authorities would have been alerted to the fact of bad transportation practice.

Whatever it was that all we Johns and Joans, Davids and Dianas, Peters and Patricias, Tims and Tammys were sublimating in a furtive touch and yet another mouth full of cow's milk fat sugar mix, it had to be something terribly different to the crude yet assumed-to-be-clean couplings of the beasts of the field, the birds of the air, the amphibians of the primary classroom's aquarium. Those hairy or slimy or feathery creatures' rutting's sole purpose was, surely the reproduction of their species. Their sexuality was most certainly not our sexuality. For we were created in the image of God and, as well, the last thing we wanted was for anybody to have a baby. It didn't matter that their tram might head off from the Collins Street and Swanston Street corner in the direction of North Balwyn or Hawthorn, or their train wind its way up along the Heidelberg line, we the earnest boys and girls of Melbourne town did not want our vaguely understood urges—our tinglings and flushings and mind wanderings—to lead to the birth process. Babies there must not be.

The animals on the other hand, wee doggies mounting wee doggies, awkwardly making the tie, tiny white mice in their cages, ever uncommunicative guinea pigs, they were on earth for the sole purpose of multiplication: there shall be wheedling puppies suckling on teats.

Among the horse folk in their jodhpurs and wellies the most intimate details of horse anatomy and horse reproduction were understood, discussed in loud voices, and if a mare had, for instance, impaction, out came the lubricant, in went the arm up the horse's bowel, mechanistically, in such a hearty and accepting-of-the-biological-realities-of-life manner that how could these dumb beasts be thought of as paralleling in their lives the lives of us, the constantly atingle with our unknowingness of sex, ice-cream eating young wasp homo sapiens?

And now that our species, created in the image of God, had learned to pasteurize the milk of cows, what harm could these brute creatures do us, being as they so obviously were, without language, memory, hope, fear; sans everything except the capacity to munch grass. Poor docile manipulable creatures with their sad eyes and their thoughtless morning and evening progress to the dairy bails, and their desireless humping, what could they be to us?

Milady's Lounge in the Athenaeum building across the street from Hilliers where the milk shakes and ice-cream sundaes were served promised our schoolgirl mating game partners more genteel facilities than did the public toilets underneath the town hall where curt messages relating to venereal disease etc, spelling out the sufferers' legal responsibilities, warned us boys of the dangers lurking inside the aforementioned girls. For us then the insideness of things was not nice.

Don't spit, it spreads TB. TB comes from the inside, from a human inside which was to us as God given and unknowable, don't-want-to-knowable, as infinity.

Milady's Lounge was run I believe by Stephanie D'Est and, if memory serves me right, Stephanie D'Est had her own radio program as well. I have always believed she came to Australia from somewhere else, a foreign place, to play the lead role in Rosemarie. She was said to rub her body in animal fat and thus preserve the lustrous beauty of her skin. But Milady's Lounge was also connected to the white slave trade. (Blond) schoolgirls, pupils of Melbourne's best ladies' colleges would enter a stall (cattle terminology) to answer a call of nature. While they were innocently controlling the function of sphincters a swarthy hand would slip under the partition dividing stall from stall, and suddenly, bingo, the blond school girl would be injected with knock-out something or other and the next thing she would know would be

Tunisia, an Arab with nothing as nice as an ice-cream sundae on his mind would be ripping off her clothes, biting at her pale flesh with his sharp white teeth.

That was in the 1950s. Later I found that there had been a parallel girl-snatching scare on the Loire in France in the 1960s: Rumour d'Orleans. There it had been believed that Jewish merchants along the Loire were luring girls into the changing rooms of their chic new style frock shops, drugging them and selling them into sexual slavery in ... North Africa, of course.

Among animals, cows are uniquely venerated, or at the very least respected, by several non-Christian cultures. Unfortunately for themselves, and for animals in general the theology of straight up and down mono-theists tends to give animals the ethical flick. There are very few animals having a good time in the Bible. In fact the only ones that come to mind are the two she bears who get to eat forty-two children because a couple of the children called a prophet, 'bald head'.

There are, however, in all religions plenty of taboos relating to what you should eat and what you should not eat. Social/functional interpretations tend to relate these eating taboos to acquired knowledge of what was healthy for you to eat. This might be simplistic, there are many possible alternative interpretations which could be put on most eating taboos. Sets of eating taboos do however tend to relate to groups of people and how those people have come to regard certain animal species. Generally eating the flesh of live animals seems pretty rare. But this might be to do with convenience. The made-in-the-image-of-God cultures pretend horror at the practice of, and most accounts of, cannibalism. Yet the nineteenth century romantic imperialist traveller among the 'primitives' is frequently self described or depicted as having some knowledge—he would rather change the subject, actually—of eating human flesh. Maybe it was just something you didn't do or talk about once you got back to the wife and kids, hung up your solar topee.

Another difficult to unravel human view of animals involves kinship with them. A whole lot of attendant taboos, eating or otherwise, follow on from this. We Scots Australians don't eat man's best friend, the dog, unless we get stuck in the South Pole that is, and even there we'd have trouble digesting collie.

I don't have room to start providing examples of this. It is interesting to note that in European societies, Christian for most of one thousand and five hundred years, there abound examples of pre-Christian animistic-to-a-greater-or-lesser-degree beliefs, atavistically embraced right up till now, particularly, interestingly enough by the arty intelligentsia—think of the last ten year's remarkable Carl Jung revival-fest.

There is enough evidence for deep-seated taboos relating to animals, to eating them, to having sexual relations with them, to having them as mad horse disease infected night mares stomping across the planes of our sleep, to terrifying effect, to make it quite clear that we cross the lines drawn by these taboos at our peril.

A lot of people sense that feeding diseased sheep's brains to cattle disrespects a taboo. In fact it plays with taboos—real or imagined—so cleverly that it seems more the plot of science fiction than part of our modern reality. Or does it?

At about the time that we, the half-made-in-the-image-of-God young of Melbourne, were ingesting milk at a rate equivalent to that at which flash and chromium embellished American automobiles were sucking up gasoline, and a hundred thousand milk bars, more, albeit of lesser social status than Hilliers, right across the state of Victoria were scooping, dripping and piping milk into the mouths of the recently and not so recently weaned, there happened upon the scene the great Australian capon scandal.

Much to the disadvantage of our feathered friends' lifestyle a stern rationality had taken a grip on the poultry industry; it had become an industry. It was at that time that several of Australia's more recent family fortunes were established on the chook's back. Packing chickens into sheds, close together, with limited life opportunity, had become all the go. There were experiments to see if they could be tricked into believing that day is night and thus increase production of eggs; their pineal glands failing to differentiate between sunlight and electric light. These new-age-for-poultry-production sheds were erected at the rural fringe of our great cities. At the same time a series of marketing boards were established to provide sinecures for the faithful, the true believers of whichever ruling political party. One of these boards' principal responsibilities was to lobby for enforced-consumption-of-the-product-they-represented legislation to ensure the growth of the industry and the transfer of as much wealth as possible from the many to the few.

Victorians approaching retirement or redundancy package age will remember the crates of milk delivered to every school in that state as part of a free milk scheme deemed to produce healthy growth in children (and to overcome fear of milk engendered in the population by the pre-vaccine incidence of poliomyelitis) but which was in fact a straightforward way of funnelling taxpayer's money into the dairy industry's production and product handling chain. In the warmer months of the year this free milk sat in crates in school yards, in the sun under peppercorn trees, curdling, setting all time highs for bacteria breeding rates. Occasionally the milk was used for milk fights. Starving students and those of limited intelligence—born to obey—drank it.

The sugar content in Australian jam was, is still I believe, guaranteed by law as a way of supporting the nation's sugar industry—I have an idea that locally manufactured jams with lower than total saturation sugar content must still be called by another name.

Back to the poor young-old capons of the story. Well, it came to pass, in urban myth and very possibly in fact, that the chicken industry discovered that you could pseudo castrate a cockerel by injecting it, in the neck, with oestrogen. A capon boom followed this great leap forward in animal husbandry. The buzz word became caponized. Come to think of it this caponization fad coincided with the opening of the first roast chicken fast food outlets. Well, as urban myth and very likely observed reality would have it the oestrogen injected into the cockerels survived the bird's turning-spit roasting at the fast food outlets.

While I don't understand the interaction between the high level oestrogen and the small quotient of progesterone in the early model contraceptive pill regime, I have often wondered if there might not be a similarity between the meaning of 'discovery' in the case of Jenner's eighteenth century partial understanding of vaccination, appropriated from 'the people' who are believed to have known about it since Roman Times, and some as yet unheralded folkloric recognition of the take-away capon, consumed in huge quantities, as a means of birth control in 1950s Melbourne.

Political realities being what they were back then, and the Catholic Church aware of its power in the state of Victoria—its principal missions being to annihilate Communism and prohibit birth control—had the contraceptive effects of the caponized cockerel been suspected, science would have been obliged to eschew the opportunity for a fast food birth control breakthrough, until community attitudes were ready for more 'sex as fun'. Whatever the reason, contraception was not declared to be the outcome of eating caponized chicken. It was believed, however, that eating these poor unbenighted-by-electric-light roasted birds caused spontaneous sex change to take place in the male of the human species; that the doses of that oestrogen which had survived cooking were upsetting the transition of the nation's boys through puberty to manhood. Manhood, an undefined property much prized in Australian society, and celebrated in that sexually ambiguous phrase 'flower of our manhood', then as now was not to be tampered with. Caponized chicken was smudging the distinctly drawn line dividing the male Australian from the female Australian. Our boys—or at least those belonging to families addicted to take-away chicken, (generally the more modern minded and forward looking)—were developing lovely breasts. Thank God, in whose image we are created, no withering of penises nor development of unwanted vulvas was actually reported in a daily press not given, in such sexually repressed times, to specific mention of the more intimate parts of the human body. Still, major changes to genitalia remained a terrifying possibility.

The Hanging Henry Bolte Victorian government of the day acted—caponizing was out. But due to better quality colour reproduction techniques, principally rotogravure, clear skin was in. The demon acne came under attack from all sides. There were proprietary acne formulations available by the score. About the time that the caponization of chickens was outlawed to save our male youth from ill defined gender characteristics; self-governed in their own interests as were milk, egg and sugar producers, and, indeed, the law, advanced thinking members of the medical profession fixed upon oestrogen tablets as the solution for boys suffering the horrors of acne. The idea was that acne was the direct result of a hormone imbalance, that a top up of oestrogen would render the facial skin as clear and smooth as that of the milkmaids so dear (or threatening, depending on your point of view) to Jenner's mind and research. Such clear skin could make the girls go for a boy and, I guess, if it came to petting they could cup the flower of Australia's youth's incipient breast in their feminine hand.

Shifting now, rather abruptly to mad cows, it has to be said that they occur in nature. Wild cattle unused to human beings are all pretty mad, or, more precisely made mad by human intervention. Dairy cows, having surrendered a great deal of their bovine separateness, handled twice daily and hand reared, tend to be particularly calm and accepting of human assistance in their lives and deaths. This could be a serious error of judgement on their part. But then it has to be argued that along with chickens and sheep, domesticated cattle have done pretty well as a species, numbers wise.

The idea 'mad cow' contains within it a whole lot of possible meanings and seems to apply to just about everything and everybody except the disease which spawned it. Certainly, amongst us homo sapiens the use of the word 'mad' has become debased with the flight of human consciousness from responsibility for the actions of the body it occupies—tricks of interpretation and elaborate reconstructions of meaning have taken language away from its natural purpose and turned it into a system of avoidance. No longer does anybody expect there to be a connection between what is said, or written, and what is done.

Mussolini: 'I've been getting reports from all over the country that the mood is overwhelmingly anti-war. I can't understand it. Industrialists, bourgeoisie, working classes, even the army, for god's sake. Yes, I know there's a deputation of artists and intellectuals waiting. What? They're going to present me with an award? Send them straight in.' From Louis de Bernieres, *Captain Corelli's Mandolin*.

When submitting to higher education, students are frequently instructed in the use of an insidious language constructed of non-meanings, non-recognitions. Increasingly, particularly in the fuzzy areas of learning, it has become accepted that the obvious, the more useful word will be substituted with one possessing more chic, even if less meaning. And there is a great deal of Greek/Roman language generated by a century of psychoanalytical practice which has legitimized itself without establishing a basis for anything of which it consists.

The camp of the sensitive-educated appears to have eliminated—with destigmatization in mind—the word 'mad' from the vocabulary we may use when talking about our own species. We no longer use it where it should be used, is needed. In truly elevated circles 'mad' may be seen no longer to exist. In its place is a plethora of terms, mostly, for the dignity of it, derived from the Latin or the Greek, which upon examination appear to represent their definitions. Upon further examination it is seen that their definitions fit the word, but no observed state of mind. One of the most outrageous of these terms is schizophrenia. Schizophrenia used to be called dementia praecox—which means precocious dementia ... which means blah blah blah. Dictionaries strive to avoid using the word mad when defining dementia, in fact mad only shows up when they translate the Latin dement. There they say dement equals mad. Mad belongs to that low order of the English language derived from German. A form of speak jettisoned by individuals striving for intellectual effect and social power. Mad belongs to the people. It is street talk. On the street everybody knows what mad means. In the Latin rhetoric of psychiatry nobody knows what schizophrenic means. It is simply a term bandied about to cover such a wide variety of behaviour types that in any other field of human endeavour except perhaps art and literary theory and culture studies, it would be abandoned. Use the word schizophrenic and it is like looking at a paddock in a mixed farm where stand sheep and cows and horses and saying look at the schizophrenics, it embraces a hopelessly wide range of characteristics.

Given this background regarding the state of language, it is interesting that Mad Cow Disease should become attached to a disease which causes the cow to display no symptoms of madness. We can use it thus, because we no longer know what mad is. There are many diseases from which human beings suffer which cause them to display symptoms similar to those exhibited by the cows suffering from Mad Cow Disease. Diseases which cause us to lose muscular and nerve control, to move in strange and unpredictable ways.

At some time in our lives most of us would have a friend who has contracted such a disease, many of us will end up suffering from such a disease, and the last thing in our minds would be to ascribe the quality of madness to a person in such a condition.

One commentator on the Mad Cow Disease scare has nominated Sad Cow Disease as his preferred alternative name for what cows would probably think of, if they could be bothered, as Mad Human Caused Disease. What we have witnessed as the media whipped up a continuing, paper selling, channel surfing, dial turning hysterical account of Mad Cow Disease is pictures of miserable animals in their death throes and the occasional spine chilling, memory provoking image of incinerators burning flesh. Having selected this item from many as the great one to run with—we must remember that there are frightening stories pouring from the world's ears and eyes and mouth every minute of the day, most of which promise at the very least, annihilation—the media has set to fudging the science, keeping unclear the likelihood of contracting CJD as a result of eating British beef.

What do we finish up with here? We have that particularly spooky, historically haunting mix of semi-science feeding hysteria while the action is underscored by ill defined notions of specificity and purity. Clearly Mad Cow Disease got up and running, in reality and in the public mind because the British government and its dud employees behaved in a power-is-everything manner common to governments and their employees everywhere, escaping responsibility while sheltering behind a screen of language and bravado. The government's people forgot to identify the meaning of the grotesque images of dying animals being blasted into the houses of its population. Images which emphasized for those who understood straight off or didn't understand that the precarious, theologically installed separation of homo sapiens from the rest of nature has always been untenable. Yet if that separation is seen to dissolve, what happens to our law, our government, our illusion of becoming?

Time now for the recounting of a fragment of a novel by Elmore Leonard. The novel was published more than ten years ago, after nine years looking for a publisher. This despite the fact that Leonard is very rich and very famous. The novel's title is *Touch*. In it a young priest receives the stigmata (if receive is the right word here) and is deeply embarrassed that this should happen. Then he discovers that he can heal people. A bunch of through and through twentieth century pragmatists get to hear of this and sniff a buck in it. Mega bucks in fact. They set up an exclusive deal where the young priest will heal a kid on prime time television. But close to the moment one of the pragmatists screws up, he has got hold of a kid with leukaemia to cure. The rest of them understand instantly that this is a big mistake because ... you can't see leukemia.

Mad Cow Disease, Sad Cow Disease, you can watch it on television, footage spliced to appear more vivid than life—or death. These tragic creatures are the beasts that suckled us indirectly through all the amazing milk bars everywhere, providing us ice-cream sundaes, milk shakes, and a school free milk to throw at our enemies, these creatures are descendants of the creatures who gave ambitious Jenner a break and kept the complexions of country milk maidens porcelain smooth. Something terrible has gone wrong with them. It might pass, it might not. Human beings may become infected, they might not. But we don't even try for a language with which we can come to terms with the problem, that is perfectly clear. Read about the disease and the language is wanting. The language is brutalized. It doesn't work any more. It is words for words' sake or covering its own arse. It is neither appropriately careless nor has it the power to identify a problem. It has deteriorated into an internalized, self-defining rant based on Latin roots and avoidance. People who single out Mad Cow Disease as a symptom of our science-technology culture's failure are just as boring, as voices, as are those determined to stone wall for the salvation of a nation's meat industry, or their own silly job with the promise of comfortable retirement.

Mad. To make mad. To make mad has, with the twentieth century abdication of responsibility from self via a number of intellectual glosses, become an outmoded notion. Before the age of psychoanalysis, over the extended period when the rural population, if not the intelligentsia knew that proximity to cows protected you from the ravages of small pox, it was believed that a fair proportion of mad people were indeed 'made mad'. We who may have made ourselves mad but can't comprehend this because the twin concepts 'mad' and 'made mad' are out of currency right now have madly thrust 'mad' on 'sad' cows and become convinced that they will infect us ... with what? Their madness or their sadness?

It is impossible to think about Mad Cow Disease without thinking of science, scientism and perceived connections between scientism and social control. As far as I am concerned social control seems to me to be the product of the humanities gone crazy if and when the humanities do go crazy and that science is rather like a school girl at

Milady's Lounge, going about her necessary business, unconscious of the language boss's controlling hand (avec syringe) moving in the direction of her edible, if not for taboo, calf muscle.

Most of the damage done to science and primary production systems (and markets) following the tardy recognition of Mad Cow Disease as a reality in the British beef herd resulted from inappropriate notions of how people should be handled—what they should be told, what they should not be told. Through the second half of this century there has been steady growth in the number of graduates in the dicey sub-science areas of psychology and sociology—the media constantly seeks and receives opinions from practitioners of these value laden disciplines—think Hugh McKay—(they love to define the conditions leading to mindless massacres or explain why lesbianism is on the rise among the educated classes, whether it is or not). It's reasonable to assume that, because of the proliferation of graduates in these areas that when something like Mad Cow Disease tosses its distressed head around government departments assuming positions in relation to the disease will be being advised by people who assume some understanding of the 'public mind'—university trained pop psychologists.

What the British government did when confronted by Mad Cow Disease was to take a psychological position vis a vis the problem. They decided to stone wall it. Mad Cow Disease, they believed, would go away. People have short memories, they thought. The people must be protected from their own tendency to hysteria.

The British government took this line because it was constructed for them in pseudo-powerful language, in proper language. In university humanities language. Nobody circumvented the crap and asked: 'What about these pictures of sad cows.'

In 1990, three years after an alert farmer had noted the disease's symptoms in his Surrey farm and been told not to publish what he had observed, the United Kingdom's Minister for Agriculture, John Gummer, tried to feed his daughter a beefburger on camera. She didn't eat the burger—evidence that she was still capable of thinking while daddy was lost in a power-language, clinging to superannuation labyrinth. I guess her position when refusing to eat daddy's on camera beef offering was akin to that of people who warn others about recreational drugs: if something might or might not be bad for you, and you don't need to ingest it, them maybe you should not ingest it.

True or false that we might catch something from eating the meat, Mad Cow Disease has all the ingredients required for a full on urban (rural) myth. The idea that there is a connection between BSE and CJD refuses to be refuted, or proved. Various statistics suggesting that there is the same or a higher incidence of CJD in countries where there does not appear to be BSE do not countermand the images of nature rendered mad. European people have come to believe that there is something very nasty in the woodshed of British agriculture. Australia's Trade Minister, Tim Fisher's, apparent delight at the prospect of the slaughter of the United Kingdom's beef herd, because that would open up a market for Australian beef producers enduring a regime of low prices, was absolutely the wrong response. Just like Mr Gummer in Britain when trying to stuff a beef burger down his daughter's throat on camera, Mr Fisher had missed the point about the images of sad cows.

People who hate science often appear strangely delighted by the disease and its promise of spreading across the species. To many of them Mad Cow Disease's existence says: That's what science does for you ... leave nature to God and God to nature. But do we want to leave God to nature? As the cleric preaches in Christina Stead's *Seven Poor Men of Sydney*:

Should you not in all functions desire only to serve god the master and return to god the fountain. The minerals do not desire to live as individuals, they stay in their colonies, sorts and orders, and accomplish their destinies, part of the common rock, although they are more beautiful than rock. Their hidden virtues do not require the sun. There are no mineral Peer Gynts. They only wish to come to the end of their foreordained cycle, to be dissolved, to crumble and enter the higher life of the vegetable kingdom and grow upwards towards the sun in green spires. The plants do not desire to vegetate; there is intense life among them, even though their existence is usually brief. They are humble, ignorant, have no voice, yet look how they are adorned when they are ripe. They put out roots, leaves, flowers, seeds, and fall to dust; millions upon millions richer than eye has seen in the jungles and wastes. They do not rebel, they accomplish their predestined cycle: but the lord has them in his hand. And if they were sentient and understood what might be their destiny even on earth, would they not give themselves up the more gladly into the maw of animals and become living flesh and blood, to see, feel, hear, have affections and praise god. Animals would certainly die joyfully if they knew they were to become part of man ... if they could understand the higher sense they would enjoy, reason, sacred love, poetry, music, and if they could have any glimmering of the soul they would inherit.

CONTRIBUTORS

Cathy Banwell is currently a researcher at the National Centre for Epidemiology and Population Health, Australian National University. She has a MA in social anthropology from the University of Auckland and a PhD in health research at the University of Melbourne. She has an ongoing interest in issues of gender and health, particularly in relation to the social construction of consumption and risk. This interest has been expressed in research on food, alcohol, tobacco, and khat.

Michael Fitzpatrick is a general medical practitioner in North London. He has written widely on the growing role of health and medical scares in the regulation of behaviour. His book *The Truth about the Aids Panic* (Junius: London, 1987) was the first to challenge the moralistic content of the British government's 'Don't Die of Ignorance Campaign' and its gross exaggeration of the danger of heterosexual transmission of HIV. He is currently working on a book entitled *The Tyranny of Health: The dangers of a primary care led NHS* which is due to be published later this year.

Simon Grant is Professor of Economics at the Australian National University. His primary field of research is in the area of decision making under uncertainty. In recent years, decision theorists have developed new models for choice under uncertainty which can accommodate the many observed patterns of choice that contravene subjective expected utility theory as well as endeavouring to be more 'realistic' or 'psychologically plausible'. In economics, this body of work has come to be known as non- (or generalized-) subjective expected utility theory.

Professor Grant's work has contributed to the development of the foundations of these theories, thereby deepening our understanding of alternative theories as well as that of the standard subjective expected utility theory.

Charles Guest is Senior Fellow, National Centre for Epidemiology and Population Health, Australian National University. A graduate of Melbourne, Deakin and Harvard Universities, he worked at the United States Centers for Disease Control, before undertaking epidemiological research in indigenous communities and, more recently, on environmental exposures, screening and disease surveillance. His interests in public health education include the communication of health topics to lay audiences and the mass media. He recently co-edited *Climate Change and Human Health in the Asia-Pacific Region* (Australian Medical Association: Canberra, 1997), and has published research and commentary in the medical and public health literature. He is currently a member of the Health Advisory Committee, National Health and Medical Research Council.

Colin Masters is Professor in the Department of Pathology at the University of Melbourne. He is one of the world's leading authorities on Transmissible Spongiform Diseases and on Creudtzfeldt-Jakob Disease in particular. He reviewed Jakob's original cases in Heidelberg and worked with Nobel Laureate Carleton Gajdusek in the 1970s. In 1979 his analysis of 1,435 cases with Gajdusek's laboratory gave one of the first global pictures of the incidence of CJD.

Iain McCalman is a Professor of History and Director of the Humanities Research Centre, Australian National University. He specializes in the history of British popular culture and politics, and has been working on dimensions of science and culture in the Romantic age. He is a member of both the Academy of the Humanities and the Social Sciences in Australia.

Hank Nelson, Professor of History, Pacific and Asian History, Research School of Pacific and Asian Studies, Australian National University. He taught for seven years at the Administrative College and the University of Papua New Guinea, Port Moresby, before shifting to Canberra. Most of his writings have been on Australian and Papua New Guinea history. Three of his books, *Taim Bilong Masta* (Australian Broadcasting Association: Sydney, 1982), *Prisoners of War: Australians under Nippon* (Australian Broadcasting Corporation Enterprises: Sydney, 1985), and *With Its Hat about its Ears: Recollections of the bush school* (Australian Broadcasting Corporation Enterprises: Sydney, 1989) were also Australian Broadcasting Cooperation radio series. His most recent book is *The War Diaries of Eddie Allan Stanton* (Allen and Unwin: Sydney, 1996). Hank has had an interest in films (*Angels of War* and *Man Without Pigs*) and has written about presenting material in different media.

Harriet Ritvo is the Arthur J. Conner Professor of History at the Massachusetts Institute of Technology, where she teaches British history, environmental history, and the history of natural history. She is the author of *The Platypus and the Mermaid, and Other Figments of the Classifying Imagination* (1997) and *The Animal Estate: The English and other creatures in the Victorian age* (1997), both published by

Harvard University Press, and the co-editor of *Macropolitics of Nineteenth-Century Literature: nationalism, imperialism, exoticism* (University of Pennsylvania Press, 1991). Her essays and reviews on British cultural history and the history of human-animal relations have appeared in a wide range of general-audience periodicals, as well as in scholarly journals in several disciplines. She was educated at Harvard University.

Robin Wallace-Crabbe is an artist, author and occasional art-writer who lives on a farm outside Braidwood in New South Wales. He has had over forty solo exhibitions since 1960 and has participated in group exhibitions of Australian art in various capitals across the globe. He is the author of four novels and an autobiography entitled *A Man's Childhood* (Imprint: Sydney, 1997), written while he was Creative Arts Fellow at the Humanities Research Centre at the Australian National University. Under the pseudenym Robert Wallace he wrote six thrillers published in the United Kingdom. For twenty years from 1970 he ran cattle in Gippsland, Victoria and in the Southern Tablelands of New South Wales. Over this period his viewpoint shifted from that of a biped to that of a quadruped.